Wild Child

A mother, a son and A.D.H.D.

by

Gail Miller

Hypatia Trust

1998

Dedication

For my son George, about whom the book is written
and for whom I have tried to do my best.

For my husband Jamie, in complete wonderment at
his 'hanging in there' and for his strong love.

For Mum, Dad and Eleanor.

For Dr. Chris Green for helping so many families
through his work.

For the Headmistress and staff of Methley Junior
School, Leeds, for restoring my faith in the teaching
profession.

Published at The Patten Press for the Hypatia Trust.
Printed and bound in Great Britain by The Book
Factory, London.

Table of Contents

NOTHing		every thing
	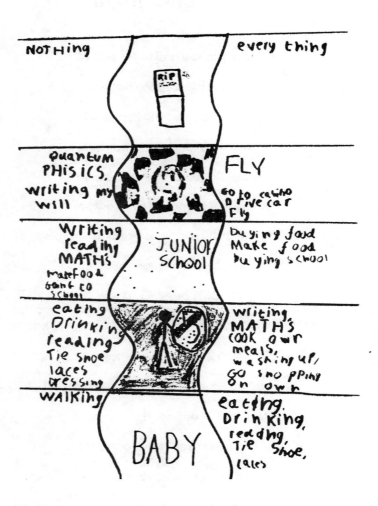 RIP	
Quantum PHISICS, writing my will		FLY go to casino Drive car Fly
Writing reading MATHS makefood gant to school	JUNIOR School	buying food Make food buying school
eating Drinking reading Tie shoe laces dressing WALKing		writing, MATHS, cook our meals, washing up, go shopping on own eating, Drinking, reading, Tie shoe, laces
	BABY	

1

Pregnancy and birth

Diary, May 1986
I am sure my period should be today. It's funny. I am usually as
regular as clockwork. If I haven't come on by tea time, then yes,
something is unusual.

My name is Gail Miller. My life has been pretty run of the mill. I attended a normal comprehensive school, took Ordinary and Advanced level exams, and then spent four years at college in Nottingham, where I had a whale of a time. I, then, came back to my hometown, met a *nice* man, married him, found myself pregnant, and this is where this book begins.

Since the start of the events I am about to recount to you, the path of my life has not been determined by me. It has been shaped by circumstances as they have happened. I am intrigued when people say 'life is just what you make it'. I have found that sometimes life just happens *to* you and you have to deal with the hand you are dealt.

If I could have foreseen events as they have occurred, I would not have let myself become pregnant in the first place. Little did I imagine how the next ten years of my life would be affected: that family relations would be stretched to breaking point, that I would be pushed to the brink of a nervous breakdown and that I would end up in a year in, year out battle with the authorities regarding this little bundle of joy to be.

Back to May, 1986. Yes, I knew I was pregnant. I had to be — and did I know it? From the realisation that it was indeed the case, I was sick with a capital S, morning, noon and night. Any food smell made me immediately nauseous. At work I spent every morning heaving over the toilet and being teased by my colleagues. I kept falling over and behaving uncharacteristically. It was as if someone else moved in to where I had been, and I was watching from the outside. One morning I fell into a crate of milk which had been delivered to work. One of the bottles broke and I cut my arm badly; though my coordination was very poor altogether, I managed to struggle on.

At twenty weeks I went for my first ultrasound scan. I would now see, for the first time, what was inside me and turning my life around. When the picture came up on the screen, I was mesmerised. The tiny foetus was waving at me. It looked really strange. Surely this wasn't right? One of its little arms kept rising up and flailing around as if trying to communicate with me. I had felt kicking at about eighteen weeks which seemed about right, but later when I was carrying my second child, I didn't feel her movements until about twenty four weeks, and believed she was different from my first born. In fact, it was actually the first born that was *different.*

I was not happy in my marriage. My husband — let's call him Bill — although pleasant at first meeting, lacked motivation, ambition or even much common sense. He was quite a lethargic person who had exhibited little ability to plan ahead, who had certain obsessive traits (and which I was later to find out were associated with the syndromes of Attention Deficit Disorder). He was so disorganised. Married to him, I became in charge of everything, from money matters to chores, to planning

8

and making sure we did things and went places. Though I wanted a companion to lean on and to support me equally, all I got was the feeling of being over-burdened. I already had one child to look after. It seemed like it was two, and that I was the 'single parent'. I suppose I imagined that this was how all married couples were, bored and frustrated with each other and always struggling just to get along.

Bill's schooldays had been, reportedly, similar to what was to come for my son Joey. He under-achieved terribly, had poor social relationships and left school unqualified. To this day his reading ability is poor and his handwriting impossible to decipher. His lack of organisation made him extremely forgetful and he couldn't concentrate for long. He was often moody. Nevertheless, he wasn't violent, quite the opposite. Bill was so 'laid back' he never argued with me about things and would not be drawn. Frequently I was frustrated because of the many unresolved issues between us.

One obsession of Bill's was his need to check things repeatedly. I have lost count of the times we were ready to go somewhere, and he would return to the house to check the electricity, or to make sure the door was locked, or something. We were always late. For one family wedding, we were running late as usual. First Bill couldn't find this, then he had to look for that. This was the normal run of things in our house. We had a mix-up with the location of the church and ended up driving round for some time before we managed to find it. Inside the service had already started and we followed the bride down the aisle to our seats.

Bill's forgetfulness infuriated me. He would go into town to get money from the cash machine, and invariably punch in the wrong number, only to have his card swallowed by the machine. This meant being left without money, without card and with great inconvenience. The solution was for me to go across town to my parents and borrow the cash until the bank opened again. Therefore, I soon assumed all the responsibility for getting the money, on top of everything else. He came home from work one pay day and couldn't find his wage packet anywhere. We were living from week to week, and without his pay, we would be unable to eat. After spending what seemed like hours looking for the money, I eventually found it stuffed down the side of the chair. I could only stand and stare, unless I let go and went to pieces in rage.

There were always a lot of do-it-yourself projects on Bill's schedule. Not only did the house look like a bomb hit it, he would either leave the work before finishing or bodge the jobs altogether. Everything was either loose or broken, and we lived with a big hole in the wall — which was going to be a fireplace — for two years. When I eventually convinced him to let me get someone in to install a new fireplace, he dropped the firefront on the brand new tiles and broke one. After waiting all that time, my beautiful new Victorian fireplace seemed ruined. His untidiness reached mammoth proportions. If I asked him to do any clearing up, he refused to put things away but would stack them in piles. He never threw anything out; the house was full of papers, old boxes, worn out clothes and old rubbish.

He took little pride in his appearance, was happiest in an old pair of jeans at least a size too big for him, full of holes and all torn and ragged around the hems. I tried throwing these old things out, but afterwards I would find them in the drawers again. He persisted in retrieving them from the bin when I wasn't looking.

It became a bit of a joke to family and friends when I described how my baby had waved at me. Perhaps we wouldn't have laughed so much if we had but known then what was in store for us all. My pregnancy progressed normally, even though the baby did move around an awful lot. I couldn't sleep at night for half the pregnancy and when I got to about thirty weeks the baby would literally somersault in my tummy all night. It is a wonder it did not choke itself with the cord.

One particular night the foetus was moving about so much that I considered calling the doctor in case something was wrong. My tummy was like a rolling ocean and the bump kept coming out in little points where the baby stuck his arm or leg out. This activity lasted for over two hours, and a couple of times I felt literally that the baby turned completely over. Even before birth Joey had an extremely high activity level. Because of this I spent the last few months in intermittent discomfort.

As my ante-natal appointments became more frequent, the nurse in feeling my tummy each time, would find the baby first this way then the opposite. As the time grew closer to the birth I suffered a bad chest infection which made me feel like death. By this time I was 'sleeping' on the couch each night because of insomnia and also the nagging Carpal tunnel syndrome which sent severe shooting pains from my wrists up my arms, expecially at night. I was also retaining fluids, so I was absolutely huge.

The delivery date came — and went. The 17th of February 1987 was the estimated delivery date, but this was later amended to 21st February, my own birthday. My stomach was now so distended you would have thought I was having twins. By the 27th of February, ante natal clinic day, I was ten days over my original delivery date, and it was decided that the baby would have to be induced. For such an active baby, he didn't show any signs of wanting to be born. He was so like his father even then. No motivation!

11

I was sent straight from the clinic into the hospital. At last! I dreamed my discomfort would be over before the night was through. Wrong! At 5pm I was given a pessary and was soon having pains in my back, but I spent a fruitless night waiting for something further to happen. First thing in the morning, I was given another pessary in the hope that it would get things moving. A nurse told me that I was in labour already, but I didn't feel contractions, just a dull ache in my back.

We waited until about 11am, when a *youth* was fetched. He came towards me with what looked like an overgrown crochet hook; this (very) young doctor tried unsuccessfully to break my waters, perhaps failing because I tensed up so much. I became hysterical, so they gave me gas and air which helped slightly to relax me. Finally he managed to pierce the sac, but only a tiny dribble of water came out. Labour would speed up now I was assured. I lay there in bed with a monitor strapped to my tummy. Apparently I was having contractions but I still wasn't feeling them. Five hours later they attached me to a drip to see if this would help speed on the contractions. By this time, I was bored with the whole thing, but at least I could sit in a chair. Two and a half hours went by with the nurse periodically turning up the drip. Finally the contractions got stronger and stronger and I was put back on the bed as the time finally came.

Eliminating the boring bits, I gave birth at 9pm after a large episiotomy to allow the baby's head smoother passage. I started to haemorrhage but the nurse pummelled my stomach and the bleeding eventually stopped. By the time the young doctor came again to put in my surgical stitches, Bill had left to find some food. Joey didn't make a sound after all that activity put up to welcome him. I felt completely let down, the big anti-climax had arrived. I even thought that through these hours I had totally lost my dignity as a woman, and certainly the privacy of my own body and emotions.

For six days I hobbled around because of the stitches, and then was discharged home.

Diary, 28 February 1987
That's it. I am never, ever giving birth again!

2

Trouble begins

My story now jumps forward to when Joey was about nine months old. Rather strangely, considering what is to follow, Joey was quite a good baby.

From the beginning he was a good eater, consuming bottle after bottle of milk. At about eight weeks we put him on the more concentrated formula milk as the ordinary type didn't satisfy him. In no time he was devouring this and I started him on solids because he was so bloated with the liquid sloshing around in his tummy. By about twelve weeks I was giving him baby rice to see if this would fill him up but soon after fed him Weetabix cereal. Once he started eating there was no stopping him. He was soon onto other, more grown up foods. His appetite was voracious but he seemed to be doing all right on it.

Joey seemed content most of the time, with only the odd bout of colic. But, once he started crying and bawling, he would go on for hours. At this time I thought this was completely normal behaviour for a baby, that all babies did this, and would give him gripe water so that eventually he would settle. I didn't know then that screaming for hours at a time was something out of the ordinary.

Diary

I wish Bill would hurry up. Joey has screamed and screamed all morning. I have tried everything to comfort him, but he wriggles and struggles when I try to cuddle him. I've been pumping milk into him like there's no tomorrow because he's so unsatisfied. He has just polished off two Weetabix and some chocolate pudding too. Could I be feeding him too much? No, I can't be, because he still seems hungry. Just what am I doing wrong?

Joey was different though, even at this early age. My daughter, who would be born some years later, was 'a piece of cake' to look after compared with him. Nevertheless, I didn't at the time find him too bad, until he got to his feet. He didn't sleep much, and found it hard to settle at night. He seemed to fight sleep and resist any efforts to settle him. But once he was walking, he turned into a tiny tornado. When Joey was about nine months of age I first shared my concerns about Joey's activity levels, and his lack of a sleeping pattern, with the health visitor.

I told her that he seemed to be on the go all the time and got into a lot of scrapes. I had to watch him at all times because he was extremely accident prone. He once wriggled so far down in the pushchair while I was hanging out the washing that he trapped himself by the neck under the bar and I thought he was going to choke. He was screaming as I tried to free him and his arms and legs were thrashing around. I managed to get him out but honestly he seemed to be able to get himself where water couldn't. This was just the start of a catalogue of accidents which were to happen, and continue to happen throughout his life.

Another time, Joey fell head first into the open coal fire while dashing around. I managed to pluck him out before he got burned, but incidents like this were regular occurrences in our house. He fell down the stairs regularly, which meant quite a few dashes to Casualty. Each time we went, we felt under suspicion because of the frequency of our visits and the fact that he was always covered in bruises. Nothing was actually said to us, but you did feel as if you were suspect due to the injuries. He could not keep still, he was into everything he wasn't supposed to be, and was generally exhausting to look after. And, with little or no night time routine, there was no relief from the everlasting feeling of exhaustion. He also had begun to have major tantrums if anything wasn't to his liking. Almost needless to say, I was getting extremely worried about him, and about my own ability to cope.

The truth is that when it is your first child causing the problems it is confusing for you. You have no other children to compare yours with. When you do try to share your concerns with other family members you get comments such as "It's the terrible twos," or "He's just boisterous" or "It's because he is a boy". You are told he will grow out of it, it is just a phase, or even that *you* are neurotic. Of course, the speaker could be right, but also may be wrong.

You carry on, hoping against hope that the problematic behaviour patterns will straighten themselves. You give it another week, then another and the weeks turn into months. Not only do the problems remain but new ones appear. When you disclose your fears to others, everyone is quick to offer an opinion on what you should or shouldn't do. The confusion persists.

15

Diary
Had the health visitor to the house again today. Joey spent the whole of last night screaming in the cot. We are trying the "checking" technique, whereby you leave the baby crying, and then go up to settle him down, first after five minutes, then ten minutes, then fifteen and so on. This emphatically doesn't work with Joey. Each evening is a nightmare and Bill and I are at a loss as to what to do next.

She didn't seem overly concerned and suggested that we just keep at it, as she tells us most babies who have trouble settling at night eventually get the hang of it. I agree, but most babies I would bet, settle down within the first hour or two. Joey is still screaming at midnight! I am going to go to the doctor and see if he can suggest anything, because I feel like I am going round the bend! When he finally does get off to sleep, I am wide awake. I feel shattered!

When you fear for the child's life because of his uncontrollable rages, when you cannot turn your back for a minute because you know he will have his finger in the electric socket or be force feeding the cat, when he is always covered in bumps and bruises because of the way he dashes about, you know something is not right. Call it gut feeling or mother's intuition, but bringing it back to myself again, *I just knew* that things were not as they should be.

Joey couldn't play properly and he was very destructive. His toys never lasted five minutes. He would throw them or break them and he couldn't stick to playing with one toy for any length of time. Everything in the toybox had to be out at once, strewn around the room. It was as if he wasn't satisfied with anything. Nothing gave him pleasure, no toy would fire his imagination. It was so disheartening for us to buy him good quality things but shortly after find them on the pile with the others discarded and useless to him. Later they would be in pieces.

Diary, 28 February 1988
Joey was one year old today. We bought him an activity centre, with lots of bells, buttons and knobs, but he was bored with it within minutes. I feel so inadequate. Bill and I pored hours over the catalogue deciding which toy would be best for him, but after all he doesn't seem to like it.

I feel so low — and trapped. Bill doesn't realise how I feel. He doesn't realise much actually. Why isn't he as worried as me about Joey? He knows that he crawls into all the most dangerous places. It is like Joey can identify everything harmful or dangerous and makes a beeline for it.

He fell down the stairs again yesterday. We are becoming regulars at the Accident and Emergency Unit. I spend all day and every day now, following Joey around and making sure he doesn't get into even more scrapes.

Within a relatively short space of time, Joey had become a complete and utter pain. He was aggressive, whinging and always on the go. I spent most of my time trying to keep him out of danger and believed that motherhood was not how it is portrayed in the parent care books.

Diary
My friend Wendy called today. She doesn't have any children, and after seeing Joey, she doesn't want any! Joey was wild, dashing up and down during her visit like a little whirlwind. Wendy tells me I look haggard. Not surprising really as I feel about 50 years old.

Bill didn't help much. He was a postman and because of the early hours he worked, he would go up to bed to have a sleep every afternoon after work. This meant that I had to try and keep Joey under control and reasonably quiet while Bill was sleeping. For Joey and me it was a daytime nightmare. We had a tiny house with a staircase running up the middle between the living room and kitchen. If I had to go into the kitchen for anything all

17

the noise which ensued drifted up the stairs and disturbed Bill. If Joey got into one of his screaming fits it was almost impossible to contain the noise and I felt under tremendous pressure to shut him up. Bill worked six days a week so this was the situation almost every day. I dreaded the afternoons because the more upset I became, the more Joey responded to it and this made him worse.

My health visitor seemed, frankly, unconcerned. I told her that Joey had turned from an angel into a monster, but she didn't grasp what I meant. I think she thought I was over-reacting and not coping well with being a mother. This was true, but Joey's behaviour was at the same time *so* challenging and my efforts at controlling him so totally ineffective that all the hassle was stopping any possibility of a close relationship between us. It was a chicken and egg situation, and one couldn't break the cycle of questions about it. I believed that there was a malfunction somewhere, but when recounting it to others, it sounded just like normal developmental stages that any child goes through.

Joey did not respond to instructions and did not learn from past mistakes. He would hurt himself doing something dangerous, and then go right out and do the same again. I was concerned, I suppose, about all the marks and bruises on him, not only for his sake, but also because people might imagine that I was hurting him. After explaining patiently to him how such an action was not a good idea, he would go out and repeat it again as if the earlier incident had not happened. By the time Joey was eighteen months old, he was quarrelsome, aggressive and didn't sleep at night. He screamed for hours when he was put into the cot. It was sheer hell!

I bought every baby magazine I could lay my hands on looking for solutions to the problems we were having. I borrowed library books in the effort to find a cause for Joey's difficulties but to no avail. These books and articles informed me that if I did A, B would happen. It could take a little while but eventually things would settle down. They didn't with Joey. What a bind parenthood was turning out to be. The health visitor promised to keep an eye on our situation. At least, my concerns were on record with her, even though she was of the opinion that it was 'terrible twos'. Little could she know that we would have terrible threes, fours, fives, sixes, sevens and eights.

Diary
I feel thoroughly fed up. I spoke to the health visitor again this week. She informs me that Joey is going through the terrible twos. Very helpful. Surely a half-blind man can see by looking at Joey that something is not right. Just look at the manic look in his eyes. He is just like an over-wound spring. And look at his skin....it's grey. Can't she see the red rings round Joey's eyes, through lack of sleep? Can't she see how exhausted I am? She thinks I am incompetent. I'm sure of it. What can't I be like Julie next door? She is coping OK.

Things got worse. Supermarket shopping was a real nightmare. Whenever Joey went into enclosed spaces like shops, he would have terrifying tantrums, and would behave atrociously, much to the amusement or disgust of other shoppers. He was always nagging for something, incessantly. He would want one thing, then something more, then something more. One item was never enough, and I did give in too often in trying to pacify him. The whole day would turn into one long argument if I didn't. Nonetheless, the *giving in* all the time reinforced the feeling of inadequacy I already felt. It was a no-win situation.

In the supermarket he wouldn't sit in a trolley, but would happily run up and down the aisles pulling goods off the shelves and sliding along the floor on his knees under other people's feet. When I tried to stop him he would scream and struggle until I just wanted the ground to open up and swallow me.

One particular day I took Joey to the supermarket and he was acting 'high as a kite'. He dashed about and wouldn't return to me, threw himself on the floor, and when I tried to restrain him, he screamed hysterically. The more I tried to contain him, the more aggressive and loud he got. People were looking on with the type of expression that every parent of a disruptive child knows and recognises. These are the faces which say "If that was my child I would give it a right good hiding" or "Look at her, why doesn't she control the little hooligan?"

In the end I got so angry and upset that I ended up screaming back at him to the horror of other shoppers. Joey got even more agitated, throwing himself round my feet at the checkout, and on and on it escalated. He got louder and the tantrum got worse. Finally I left the trolley there full of shopping, smacked the living daylights out of him and vowed never again. Oh, the amount of times I was to say "never again" in the coming years! That was, in fact, the last time Joey went into a supermarket until he was about six and a half years old. I started dropping Joey off at Mum's whenever I had to go shopping. It was just so much easier to let Mum look after him when I went out and did whatever was necessary. That arrangement carried on for some years, and I was lucky indeed to have this possibility.

When Joey was between the age of two and three years, I had consulted the family doctor, regarding the difficulties I was having with all aspects of Joey's development. The issues I was most concerned about were, of course, his impulsiveness leading to frequent injuries, and the fact that we couldn't get Joey into any sort of bedtime routine no matter how hard we tried.

Although I again got the 'terrible twos' lecture, the doctor reluctantly agreed to give Joey some sedative medicine to see if this helped. Joey was often still awake and active at 11pm and later. Not the best state of affairs for any of us.

Diary
The doctor prescribed some medication to help Joey settle down at night, but he has been taking it a week now and he is thriving on it! It is not having the slightest effect. I am still up and down stairs all night. Maybe I am making Joey like this? Why is he so crotchety with me? Am I doing something to him, or giving him something which is not agreeing with him?

Mum doesn't help. She keeps saying that you need a lot of patience when you have children. Tell me something I don't know! She makes me feel like an inadequate Mother though, with her comments. I feel helpless and hopeless. The girl next door had her son Jason, the month before me. She is only nineteen and Jason is so placid. She is coping fine with motherhood. What is wrong with me?

The medicine was Phenergan. Unfortunately for us it had no effect whatever in helping Joey calm down at bedtime, but it did make it difficult for us to rouse him in the mornings. Finally Phenergan was abandoned, and my long and unfruitful relationship carried on with the health visitor.

Diary
I hate my life. Friends have stopped visiting because of all the chaos and mess. Joey is running me ragged, and Bill is just — well, Bill. I feel a failure as a mother because I just cannot get close to Joey. I don't like him. I sometimes wonder if I brought the wrong baby home from hospital, but I know in my heart he is mine, and he is the image of bill. Just a little clone, right down to the flat bit on his right ear. Bill has one of those too!

This isolation is a killer. Some days I want to just pack my things and get out of this place. What would happen to Joey then?

21

Could I really leave him if it came to the crunch? What am I thinking of? I am intelligent and have a degree! Why do I feel such a wreck and why can't I think straight? I would feel better if someone could just understand. Mum has Joey for me now and again so that I can get a break, but she cannot see anything wrong. Surely I am not imagining Joey's difficulties?

What about the health visitor and doctor....aren't they supposed to be experts? I just cannot accept that Joey's tantrums, and activity levels are normal. I feel it in my bones. There IS something wrong, I know it! No one believes me though. What do I have to do to get my point across?

3

Three Years Old

Joey grew more and more into his odd behaviour, and showed no signs of growing through or out of it. My Mum and I started taking him to playgroup, but even there with all the other boisterous toddlers, Joey still stuck out like a sore thumb. He dashed around knocking others off their feet and couldn't play normally. His manner to other playmates was very aggressive and unfortunately lost him potential little friends.

He always came home covered in bruises. He fell off gym equipment, launching himself off benches, and so forth. He had no sense of danger or consequences. One morning Mum took him to playgroup to give me a few hours off, but returned home very distressed because Joey had climbed onto a high table, fallen off and cracked his head. By the time they got home a great lump had come up on his forehead. There was, of course, nothing she could have done to prevent it.

It became obvious that even amongst the most boisterous of kids, Joey was different - more aggressive, more over the top in everything he did. He never talked, he shouted. Instead of walking with me, he dashed off down the street while I ran after calling and pleading for him to stay near. He was more than a handful, rather like having a devil in the house. His erratic and completely unreliable response to all manner of situations worked its destruction on me as well. I continued feeling extremely sorry for myself when comparing my situation with that of other mothers, many much less educated than I, but coping with a whole gaggle of children who were no bother whatsoever. Why did I end up with a child like this? Why was bringing up one child too much for me?

Mum decided that perhaps a nursery school would take care of some of his surplus energy, whereas the playgroup was only that, a playgroup and not a school. Fortunately there was a nursery quite near to us and they agreed to take him for mornings only. Strangely, this seemed to work reasonably well. Joey would get up out of his seat at inappropriate times and wander around the classroom; this may have been disconcerting to the teacher at the time but didn't cause major problems. Then after a while he did full days. Although this period in nursery school was relatively uneventful for Joey, he was still naughty and uncooperative at home.

Bill and I weren't getting on well at all. I was frustrated with him because of the way he was, and because he didn't seem to have any idea of how I was feeling about the strained relations between us. Some days I hardly spoke to him, but he never asked why I was acting in that way. He buried his head 'in the sand' about everything so we never discussed anything, and issues were never resolved.

Diary
I have decided. I am leaving. I don't know when. I don't know
how, but I am going to do it. If I carry on like this I am going to
end up in the mad house!

Nor could Bill see the links between his own childhood and Joey's. He had himself a terrible time at school, finally leaving at 14 with no prospects and no motivation to change anything. Only recently did I learn from his family that he had been sent to a 'special school' in the end, because of his problems. It is too easy to say now, but if only Bill had warned me about the extent to which his own childhood had been marred, I might have thought twice about conceiving.

Ultimately I just couldn't go on living with him. He was a very nice man who didn't have a bad word for anyone, but we proved not at all compatible. Living in the tight circumstances of a terrace house, crammed to the brim with hoarded rubbish and little money, here I was in my late twenties feeling that my life had finished already. I became badly depressed, and the depression was greatly exacerbated by Joey's behaviour. Life became such a blur that I can barely recall the detail.

My thirtieth birthday arrived and this was the catalyst that spurred me on to change my situation. While knowing that it would be difficult for me on my own with Joey, I told Bill I wanted a divorce. He said little and didn't contest it. Joey was three years and five months when the divorce came through. I had custody of Joey, though Bill has always seen him twice a week up to this day. Subsequently he has always paid maintenance for Joey, and our relationship since the divorce has been completely amicable. I stayed with my parents temporarily while trying to get things sorted out. These few months proved a revelation, and a frightening one, especially for my now retired parents, who saw their quiet home turned into a madhouse.

Of course my parents knew, by this time, that Joey caused problems, but when we moved in with them, it became clear how extreme Joey's behaviour had become. Even though his unruly behaviour was there for all to see, the reactions differed between Mum and Dad and wreaked havoc on their own relationship as well. On the whole Mum denied there was a problem, and Dad thought Joey was a brat who I had let get away with murder. Mum believed that my divorce had caused the problems that arose, but since his behaviour only continued as before, this analysis didn't help.

One day Joey got hold of a piece of plastic curtain track and while I was trying to remove it from him, he jabbed it directly into my eye. I was hurt, of course, and he had managed to cut into the tender skin under my eye. He thought this was a real hoot of a game, but I wasn't laughing. I gave him a smack, but Mum stuck up for him, saying he hadn't done it on purpose. I knew he had, but he just hadn't seen the consequences of his actions: he could not realise that poking someone in the eye would hurt.

There were numerous incidents like this, and many disagreements surfaced between my parents. I couldn't agree with either of them in fact. I had done my utmost to look after Joey to the best of my ability. I had disciplined him, tried to teach him right from wrong and explained about appropriate and inappropriate behaviour. This had not affected him, or sunk into his understanding of where he was or who he is. I tried to explain the situation to others by saying, "there is *the* world, and there is Joey's world. These are two almost separate places." This was the best way I could describe things. Joey was out on a limb and out of step with others. It wasn't an external thing, I was sure of it by this time. There was something in Joey that made him this way. Helping other people to understand this was another matter.

Diary
Joey and I moved into our house this week. The divorce went through without a hitch. I now will have to carry the burden alone. If you look at the other parents in the street or at the school gates, they don't have these problems. What have I done to deserve this purgatory?

Joey has begun to indulge in lots of thrill-seeking behaviour. My heart is in my mouth when I see some of his antics. At the moment he is again covered in bruises. He is also doing really weird things with his belongings. The other day I found three pairs of soiled underpants hidden under his mattress. Why is he doing such strange things?

I feel so exhausted. He is really hyperactive today. First he wants to play in water, then he puts the television on and watches something for....all of five minutes. Then he wants to play with with the cushions, but when I let him do it he hurts himself. He goes outside for a little while, is soon bored and in again. He is trashing the place too. He goes mad if I tell him he cannot have something. He has broken so many things and has no conception of value. His temper just takes him over and woe betide anything or anyone who gets in his way.

I have stopped taking him out with me. It is just not worth it. I see the looks on others' faces when he throws himself around, or hits me in public. Let's face it, he is a little brat. Obnoxious in fact. I am going to have to see the health visitor again, not that she can do anything, but at least the record will go on about the problems here!

4

School & Joey

Joey's difference went public, so to speak, when he moved up from nursery into primary school. He was intelligent enough. In fact, subsequently he was found to be way above average intelligence. Equally however, he was far in front of everyone else for being always in trouble.

He couldn't sit in his seat long enough to participate in class work and was excessively active in his wanderings around the classroom at inappropriate times. He nagged and interrupted until he drove teachers to distraction. Some handled him better than others, but slowly and surely he was becoming labelled as 'troublesome'.

There were certain other children to whom Joey always seemed to gravitate — and this has always happened all the way through school — and these were not a good influence on him. He was irresistible to children who were disruptive, or who were easy to wind up like himself. Together they were always in trouble. We told Joey to keep away from particular classmates but he was like a magnet to them. The more teachers tried to keep them apart, the more the attracted each other. Often Joey also picked up blame for the activities of other children, which first spawned his belief that he was being picked on and victimised. By now, all the negative reactions from others, myself included, began to take their toll. His own self esteem and pride first started to dwindle in the school situation.

Diary
I could not leave the house today. I have had a particularly bad time with Joey this week. My confidence has totally gone. I certainly did not see a life like this for myself ten years ago! What happened to that carefree fashion student? She was in another life, another place and time.

I am a bad mother. Joey dislikes me, and I him. when I look at him sometimes I imagine whether or not it would be worth the risk of trying to get rid of him. In my worst moments I imagine my fist crashing into his little face, and it crumbling under the blow. His teeth click together and I hear and feel the bones break. You little bastard. You have ruined my life for sure. I am trapped in a living hell, from which I see no escape. Could I arrange it so that one of his accidents is fatal? Would I be able to get away with it? Would a life in prison be preferable to this life I am trapped in? At least I would get some peace!

At four and a half, Joey contracted encephalitis, a serious viral brain infection, and we nearly lost him. This occurred in the summer holidays when he had only been at school full time for a few weeks. He had been out of sorts for a couple of days, but had gone out with his Dad at the weekend. The next day he appeared ill so I called the doctor who diagnosed a virus and gave us paracetamol. Joey didn't improve so I called the doctor back in the afternoon, and after seeing him he immediately rang the hospital. I was told to take him straight there. Joey went downhill fast as his limbs stiffened and his skin went a funny blue colour. We found out afterwards that they had given him only a 50:50 chance of recovery. Lots of tests were done on him such as lumbar puncture, EEG, ECG and ultrasound scanning. After five days in hospital he had a fit and went into a coma in the middle of the night. A rash came up under his armpits and slowly spread to other parts of his body. Up until this point the staff had been stumped for a diagnosis, even bringing in a paediatrician who specialised in tropical diseases through Joey had never been abroad, or even further than the next town.

Thankfully Joey did regain consciousness and was then rushed to another hospital in a nearby town where he was put on an infusion of strong antibiotics. Mercifully he began to improve. Further tests revealed that Joey had a meningitis type illness. Encephalitis was diagnosed and we were informed that a virus had got into Joey's brain. It remained to be seen whether or not he would be left permanently impaired. He was having hallucinations by this time and his speech was rambling, but after about nine days he began to eat again. The hospital staff who were tending to Joey were overjoyed when he started to recover. He had been in the hospital for quite some time and there were nurses who had become quite attached to him. Though his recovery had begun, he was not wholly well. When he came home he was rather like a little stick insect. The loss of weight, the blue tinge to his skin, his weakness overall were pitiful, but the really big change was that the hyperactivity had gone. He stayed off school for about a month in order to gain some weight and convalesce.

When he did return to school, everyone was really nice to him. The teachers made allowances for him because of the trauma he had been through. But how things changed when he regained his strength again. As he improved physically, the giddiness, impulsiveness, lack of concentration and insatiability re-emerged, only ten times worse.

Some little time later, Joey went back to the hospital for tests of brain function and possible impairment. He took the Wechsler pre-school and primary scale of intelligence, which examined a number of different skills such as mazes, number tests, copying patterns with blocks, comprehension, and he did extremely well. At the end of the tests, completed over two days, the psychologist informed us that Joey found the tests for his own age too simple, so she had carried on testing him with questions for older children. He had flown through these with flying colours. She considered at that time that Joey was well above average intelligence. Superficially there was no impairment from the illness; his report follows:

Pontefract Health Authority, Clinical Psychology Department, 9 December 1991

From the Clinical Psychologist to the Consultant Paediatrician, **Re:Joey Miller. 28.2.87**

Further to the letter from SH dated 19th September I have arranged to see Joey in order to complete the subtests of the Wechsler Pre-School and Primary scale of intelligence (WPPSI) to assess his level of cognitive functioning. He completed subtests of comprehension, geometric design and block design and performed at a level well above that expected of a child his age. **I am now able to confirm that Joey is a very bright little boy whose cognitive functioning remains superior despite his illness.** His mother and grandmother said they have no concerns about his general level of performance and thought he was back to his normal self. [Signed.]

My questions are many. If Joey is so intelligent why should he underachieve so severely in the following years? Why would he fail so miserably socially and end up with no friends? Why would teachers and classmates dislike him so much? Why would he suffer all the pain and heartache that was to come? As time went on, his behaviour continued to cause major problems for him both at home and at school. I consulted the health visitor again but she could offer no real assistance.

One avenue that she suggested seemed a possible way forward. She suggested that perhaps he was hyperactive due to the foods he ate. Her opinion was that we should try cutting certain foods out of his diet over a period of time, eliminating anything which we suspected might be making him 'high'. When you are in a plight such as we were, you are desperate for *any* solution to the problem, so we set about this task with gusto. Because we could not get an appointment with a dietician, we decided to initiate and supervise the task ourselves. I read up on everything I could find on the subject, and it all seemed to make sense to me. You are what you eat. Perhaps we would be able to temper Joey's problems by adjusting his diet?

A variety of things were suggested as possible culprits in his diet. First we stopped the eating of anything coloured such as oranges, brown bread, gravy and the like. We knocked out things with a wheat content, then milk, fruit, eggs, cola, smarties, and chocolate. You name it and we tried to eliminate it for enough time to see a benefit. But it appeared that adjustments to Joey's diet had no effect on him whatsoever. It was so upsetting to stop something, be looking for any improvement in his behaviour, and have our hopes raised when he might have a good day, or even a couple of hours. When his behaviour deteriorated as it inevitably did, it was really heartbreaking. Whatever could we do next? Naturally I am pleased to hear of parents who cut out certain foods from their children's diet and get 'miraculous' results. Because of our experience I am by no means convinced. I would love for it to have worked with Joey, but it just didn't.

I wrote to the Hyperactive Society, asking for their information, hoping that this might shed light on why adjustments to Joey's intake made no difference. It appeared we had done more or less the right things, by eliminating one food at a time to see if it helped. Nevertheless, in our case it had not. The Society's leaflet offered another hope for some hyperactive children, and this was that Evening Primrose Oil, either taken orally or rubbed into the skin, might have beneficial effect. We tried it; every morning and evening I rubbed down the insides of Joey's arms.........but again, with no effect.

More time passed, and for me the bizarre and incomprehensible behaviours that Joey exhibited were maddening in the extreme. My relationship with Joey was shot to pieces. I disliked him intensely and wondered what I was doing to make him behave this way. He got more aggressive, angry, and frustrated by the day. He had a vile temper and a real attitude problem, stomping about and throwing things in his rage.

Sometimes we wondered if he was just being awkward. For example, if you asked him to go get his socks on and to bring a book whilst he was at it, he would either do one of these things, neither of these things, or go off and do something completely different. It was as if the messages were blocked, or jumbled between his ears and his brain. He picked up and understood fragments of what was being said to him, but not all. In years to come we would discover that this was the way his brain worked and we had to accommodate to that in order to reach him, but at the time we simply got frustrated and angry. Even to this day I hate myself for it.

Diary

Joey has been impossible today. He has snapped and bitched at me all day, and he won't do anything for me. He refuses point blank to follow instructions. I tell him a hundred times a week to get his jumper on the right way, instead of back to front, or to put his shoes on the right feet. You would think by the law of averages that he would them on the right feet at least 50% of the time wouldn't you, but no, not Joey.

Some of the younger kids are dressing themselves completely by now, but Joey gets everything muddled. I even caught him with his pyjamas on over his daytime clothes the other week. Is he just lazy, or is he doing these things to get at me, or to drive me insane?

I feel sure this child hates me. I try my best, but it is really hard. Why do I have to keep repeating instructions over and over again? Why won't he learn from his mistakes? What am I doing wrong?

A major problem was his inability to concentrate for more than a few seconds at a time. His mind and body were all over the place. You could not play a game with him, read a book to him, sit him down to watch a television program, or make him understand normal rules and instructions. He could not stay in one place long enough for any of these normal activities. His troubles at school were unabating, and shockingly he began to use swear words that you would not credit from the mouth of a five year old. I imagined that the school thought Joey lived in a real madhouse, with no rules, no discipline, and a mother with a colourful and wide ranging vocabulary of the most unsocial kind. Joey was not getting the swear words from me or his home. They must have come from the school yard itself, and other children.

Whereas so-called normal children could differentiate when to use this language and when not to, i.e. when teachers were not in earshot, or when it would not get them into trouble, Joey could not. His impulsiveness never allowed him to hold back under any circumstance. Naturally this did not appeal to the sensibilities of listeners. Joey gave the impression of having no respect for authority, be it teachers or parents. Because of this, others thought that he had a discipline problem. Naturally I did not like being shouted and sworn at by him either, and it was absolutely discouraged by me. I tried smacking Joey for his misdemeanours, reasoning, rewarding, shouting, bribing, negotiation, you name it. Nothing worked or even stemmed the tide of his overwhelming performance. He carried on charging through life like a little roadrunner with no regard for others who he knocked over on the way.

He took pleasure in nothing. After whinging and nagging until he got what he said he wanted, he wanted it no longer. He was straight on to the next thing, then the next. He couldn't work toward rewards and everything had to be immediate. He was like an over-stretched elastic band, always ready to snap. If something did not go his way his anger didn't rise in degrees. He would just flip at the slightest thing. It was really frightening to watch. When he got like this it reminded me of that television program, *The Incredible Hulk*, where the hulk would burst out of his shirt, and turn from a man into a big angry green monster. Joey was just like this. You could see the blue veins come up on his neck as he threw himself round in a blinding rage.

Since he was just like a pressure cooker waiting to blow, it was difficult to know what to do in these situations. There was no calming him when he was thrashing, and if he caught me off-guard, it could really hurt. I usually tried to calm him with words, but it was extremely difficult to stay calm myself.

Joey was so unfair in his approach and attitudes to daily life. He was, and still is, totally self-centered. He had no ability to grasp how his actions were impacting on others around him, and appeared to have no regard for other points of view. Hence, there was no explanation which could reach him as to how his actions were not acceptable in this society, or how he was hurting others.

His reputation at school was black indeed. Other parents warned their children to keep away from him because *he was trouble*. This really hurt me, and also hurt me for him. I understood how other parents felt, how they worried that their own children might be harmed,

A mother, a son & ADHD

either purposefully or accidentally. Trust it to be my kid who is the one rapidly gaining a reputation!

5

A catalogue of daily life

At the risk of being overly-repetitious, I think it is important for the readers of this account to know some of the gory details of Joey and his life. It may help another parent to understand the behaviours and actions of their disruptive child, even though little is understood clearly about the origins of this set of conditions which have come to have labels in the medical world, even if temporary ones. Any reader will also realise that inevitably as author, my own analysis is interlaced with the actual behaviours of Joey and what I report is as honest as I can be in the circumstance of suffering along with him. Mother and child are bound, of course, but also separate individuals. In the circumstances I am describing and observing the child, with little or no consciousness of even being 'seen' in return, let alone observed by my son.

At his primary school, Joey consistently challenged every rule, and was a thorn in the side to all his teachers. He became a class scapegoat because of his disruptive tendencies. He got into trouble for the things he did, but he also collected other children's blame and their teachers' irritation along the way.

This tore his self esteem, his pride, to shreds. He began to believe he was bad. It is actually the things he did that were sometimes bad, but a child of such a young age finds this distinction hard to make. And, it is sometimes quicker and easier to blame a problem child than to get to the bottom of a situation. Admittedly, a child such as Joey becomes involved in numerous disturbances at school, but he was in fact not often the instigator.

He could not foresee the consequences of his actions. If a classmate called him a name, Joey would lash out, firstly because of his highly-strung nature, and secondly, because he recognised no outward reasons — like a teacher, or a code — why he should not respond immediately. He would get caught easily, and punished, and the instigator, likely as not, would leave him in it without looking back. This happens time and again, so that eventually the disruptive child becomes a self-fulfilling prophesy. Sometimes Joey knew he wasn't responsible for starting the trouble, but he hadn't the means of communication and appropriate response mechanisms to put this across to the teachers. Because of this lack, the child lashes out either verbally or physically, and cannot be tolerated in a classroom environment under normal circumstances. It is easy to see how expulsion or exclusion actually occurs.

The type of scenario described above happened often with Joey. He was put under a great deal of pressure due to certain characteristics, for example, not being able to concentrate and not being able to sit still. He attracted the wrong sort of children as friends, those who were attracted by the excitement of conflict, and therefore was frequently in trouble because of incidents in which they all participated. All of this was in his school day, and on top of the trouble he was into at home. The burdens of this pressure were too much for him to bear.

I became a regular at the headmaster's office. In fairness, however, the school had a very kind and experienced headmaster, one who was concerned without condemning us in any way. He wanted to help

36

us. Whenever there was an incident, I would go in, solutions would be suggested, and put into operation. Sadly, nothing changed. Joey was definitely being hampered by something.

One concern expressed by the Headmaster was the way that Joey seemed to switch off in class as if he lost consciousness momentarily. Was he having fits, or did his ears need testing? If he had a hearing impairment this might account for his staring into space for short periods, the switching off, lack of attention and the flitting from one thing to another. If he couldn't hear what the teachers were saying he would do things like this, and deafness might explain all his other problems. But, this was not the case.

Diary
Mum is on at me again. Joey has been in trouble at school, but once again she is insinuating that they are just tormenting him. I know that he doesn't get a fair chance sometimes, but he is usually involved whenever there is trouble. Why can't she understand that we aren't doing him any favours by standing up for him at all costs. Surely this is showing him that it is all right to swear at teachers, or kick chairs around the classroom?

Joey's ever-present bumps and bruises were the result of a combination of accidents and self-inflicted injuries. He bumped into things, dashed rather than walked and tripped up due to poor coordination. One of his favourite tricks was zipping himself up in a sleeping bag and throwing himself down the stairs repeatedly. He had skin burns on his back where he had hit himself on the edges of the steps. If I tried to stop him, he might stop briefly, or have a tantrum, then when the coast was clear, he would return to do the same thing again, pleading "just one more, just one more". In situations like this, it seems easier to allow the child to do

37

something dangerous, rather than risk the trouble and strife that arises in attempting to control it.

There is also sometimes the creeping feeling (however dreadful this may sound) that perhaps the child will kill himself in the process, and you will be free. I know clearly what is meant by the epigram, 'anything for a quiet life'. I lived with constant quibbling, nagging, questioning, hyperactivity, arguing and oppositional behaviour. Remember this is day in week out, month in year out. Only another parent with such a child can understand the absolute hell on earth, and constant torment of living like this.

Diary
Joey's nagging has been really getting me down lately. He thinks I am a bottomless pit. He wants more, more, more! I have spent a fortune recently on toys for him, to see if anything will inspire him. Why can't he be like other children? I see kids every day playing in the street with a tea towel round their head, or a sheet for a cape. They play at pretend for hours, but I have never managed to get Joey to engage in pretend play. He just wants to destroy things.

He got through twelve bottles of juice this week. The boy's thirst is unquenchable, and why is he always so clammy? Sometimes I recoil when I touch him, he is so sticky and wet. I feel so detached from Joey. I want to love him, but there's nothing there to love. He is abusive to me, will not go along with any of the house rules, and his constant clamouring for attention, positive or otherwise is draining me. I look at him sometimes, just willing him to understand what I am trying to tell him, but it is no good. He either can't or won't cooperate.

Joey had a penchant for bouncing, somersaulting and jumping off the bed. He also liked to climb on top of high things and jump. Apart from all the little scratches and bruises he invariably had, he always had one major injury on the go, be it a bump on the head, a cut, a large bruise, or something. He seemed impervious to pain. It was as if he enjoyed being hurt. Repeatedly he took all the foam cushions off the sofa, piled them up and got on top, teeter-tottering to keep his balance then falling, banging his head or hurting himself in some way. Did he take any lessons from this? Not likely! He would repeat the exercise again, thriving on thrills, foreseeing no dangers, processing no retainable information. It was no use explaining the dangers of certain actions to him. I tried innumerable times with no effect whatsoever.

But not only dangerous or daring things were on Joey's agenda. Sometimes he was simply acting in a ridiculously stupid way which remains inexplicable. I was still on my own with Joey at this time, and between visits to the health visitor I was dealing with everything on my own. Dad had no time for Joey, and Mum was a dead loss; she simply blamed me for the situation. She would probably deny it now, but this is how I felt. One evening at about 8pm, Joey came to me saying that he had Lego up his nose. I laughed, thinking it was one of his wind-ups as he has always been a bit of a clown on top of it all. Nevertheless, on inspection, yes, there it was. A Lego light jammed up one of his nostrils. He must have pushed it well in because it was so high up that I couldn't reach it. Off we went to Casualty and the amused, and probably bemused, nurse managed to get the offending Lego out with a scissor type implement. Joey whinged and screamed all the way through the procedure, and I couldn't help thinking, yes, you're sorry now "until the next time!"

Thinking that it might fire his imagination, I bought Joey a computer. He had nagged and nagged for one and he had always been into technical things so I hoped it would help. His interest lasted for about four months if that. Finally all the program cassettes ended up with the tape pulled out, strewn over his bedroom and in various other hiding places. I was tidying his room one day when I came across the computer, and noticed that the keyboard looked strange but I couldn't figure out why. Looking at it carefully, I realised that all the letters were in the wrong places. On questioning him, but not before much denial, Joey admitted he had hit it with a baseball bat. The keys had come out with the battering and he had tried to replace them so that I wouldn't know.

Joey always denied his misdemeanours, and still does. He destroys something, messes up a room (say the bathroom, by scattering talc and bubble bath all over the place) but never admits it was him. He cannot grasp that if I know I had not done it, then it had to be him. This concept was totally alien to him: he somehow believed that as long as he denied something — even to the bitter end — that would become reality.

Also in this period when we were still on our own, Joey began engaging in weird ritualistic actions and harbouring strange obsessions. He began hiding things. He rolled clothes up into tight little balls, and stuffed them in out of the way places. He hid dirty clothing, so that items of his attire would mysteriously vanish. I had to look all over the house to find things to wash. I tried to drum it into him that dirty washing should be put in the wash basket, so that it could be regularly cleaned. I believe my explanations were logical: a good habit is to take responsibility for your own things, a good thing is to have clean clothes for school on a daily basis, if dirty clothes are hidden away they cannot get washed, it is bad (inconsiderate) to have Mum distressed all the time when she cannot find clothes that have been hidden, this is really improper and inconsiderate behaviour. As a last resort, *if it happened again he would get a smack*.

No explanation or threat had any effect on him. He went on hiding things as if he was deaf. I really did not know what on earth to do with him. He just seemed

40

to get worse and worse and *worse*. His main obsession was about underpants. If he soiled them ever so slightly, there was a much greater chance of him hiding them. He found the most obscure places to conceal them, and sometimes I found them in the waste bin. He could not tell me why.

By now my parents, Harold and Mary, knew that I was having extreme difficulty in being a parent to Joey. They had known, of course, of the troubles with him from a very early age, but too much at a loss to know how to deal with the situation, or give me considered advice. It was clear that Mary felt my parenting was to blame for Joey's problems. She could not however give positive suggestions. Harold openly stated that Joey did not get enough discipline and this was the problem. I *had let him get away with things*, and had not been firm enough when he was little. In reality, however, the opposite was true. Joey was disciplined more than other children. He needed *more* consistent boundaries because he challenged *more* boundaries than other children.

Diary
Mary feels I should stand up for Joey even when he is in the wrong. Is that the right way to go about things? I don't know. When she says things like this, she really diminishes my confidence in my own decisions, and I don't know whether what I instinctively feel about a situation is right or not. I am pulled in opposite directions, and feel so unsure all the time. Between them, they have got me to a state where I don't know if I am right or wrong. Mum always takes the opposite stance to me, and I feel like every decision I make is the wrong one. My head is bursting!

The trouble was though, that after years and years of this thing wearing away at me, and after trying every disciplinary technique with no effect, I had also begun to believe that it was my lack of parental skill which produced a 'wild child'. Outwardly , I looked the

41

ineffective parent bringing up a very naughty child, therefore the explanation is that the child is naughty because of one's own disciplinary style and lack of skill.

Mary thought, and still does, that the sun shone out of Joey's backside. Because of all the aggravation he had at school she got into the way of thinking that everyone else in the world was wrong and Joey was the only right one. It was true that he was being persecuted, that he was frequently involved in negative incidents, and that he definitely displayed the behaviours which caused him further problems at school. But she would not admit that Joey's behaviour was in any way challenging. She thought the teachers and I were not patient enough with Joey. She believed I did not give him enough attention and that those at the school were tormenting him.

Diary
Joey has wrecked his bedroom this week. I spend so many hours a week clearing up after him and sorting his chaos out for him, and he still does this! I have spent most of the week in tears. Has any other parent every given birth to such an ungrateful, uncaring, unfeeling little brute? Last week he scattered talcum powder all over the bathroom and it took me over an hour to clear up the mess. What did I find when I went back into the bathroom? The same again, but this time with lotion smeared over everything. The child is destructive to the extreme. I cannot, at present, think of one redeeming feature about his personality, and I detest him for the hell he is making of our lives. At the same time I really feel for him. Surely he doesn't like being forever in trouble? Why has he got to make me suffer like this though? Does he enjoy seeing me so upset?

I have been getting a tight pain in my chest lately. I'm finding it difficult to breathe. Perhaps I should go to the doctor.

Attention, in fact, close attention was what I was giving him. I was giving him so much that I was exhausting myself. He would flit about from one thing to another, trailing destruction behind him. My life had become one long round of clearing up after him, trying to mend things he had broken, keeping him out of danger when he would insist on trying to *kill* himself, and attempting to satisfy his hunger and thirst. He was voracious in this respect. He ate and ate, and be in and out of the fridge all day. If he couldn't have what he wanted he would either have a tantrum, or steal it. His thirst was unquenchable. He drank and drank, and was always hot and clammy from all his dashing about. It was just more, more, more — more food, more toys, more attention.

Mary believed that Joey would grow out of it (a four year long story by then): it was because he was bored or because I was divorced, or because.... Everyone seemed to have an opinion, but no practical help to offer. Joey was five by then and his odd compulsions increased. Apart from hiding things, he got into the habit of taking his duvet out of its cover each night. This really infuriated me because it is so hard trying to get those stupid things into covers anyway. Having to replace it each morning was maddening, and Joey could give me no explanation. He also went through a phase of sleeping under his bed instead of on it, or sleeping with his head at the foot of the bed. These obsessions came on top of the behaviours already there but did not replace them; these were add-ons. There seemed no end to the peculiar traits the child could amass. As time went on, I got more frazzled, Joey seemed to get more of the devil in him, and I was rapidly arriving at the point where I couldn't take much more.

Diary
Joey got out of bed in one of his moods — again. I have had such a bad day today that I could willingly walk out of here and never come back. I don't know if I have the courage to kill myself. Joey wears me down with his constant bickering, whinging and arguing, and he changes like the English weather. One minute he

is alright, and then he flips. He is like a Jekyl and Hyde character. No wonder I am always on edge. Recently the palpitations in my chest are really worrying.

6

New Start: New Life?

In 1992, when Joey was five, I met the man who was to become my second husband. His name is Simon and when it looked like he was going to be permanent in my life, I introduced him to Joey. From the beginning Simon was appalled at what a little monster Joey was. It was shocking to him that a five year old could be so moody, belligerent and aggressive. This was the first time he had met a child like this. (Later through my work with the support groups, he would learn that about one in twenty children suffer from ADHD to one degree or another.) In fairness, Joey's behaviour *was* really bad, and getting worse. He wanted all the attention, positive or otherwise. He didn't concentrate, was impulsive, frustrating and altogether an enormous challenge.

Simon came into our lives with no children of his own and no parenting experience. In addition he had been in the Air Force, so was keen on routine, discipline and structure. Imagine how he saw us! There I was with a child who ruled our roost, who threw a tantrum to get his way, who did no wrong according to his grandmother, and who never adhered to normal routine or instruction. Inevitably the family situation became inflamed.

Instead of me being encased in the middle of a triangle with Mum, Dad and Joey pulling at each corner, I was now in a square with Simon at the fourth corner. I was becoming weaker as the days went by, torn in all directions by the arguments in the family regarding the way Simon tried to deal with Joey. He smacked him which didn't sit well with Mum. Not really with me either because I had stopped smacking Joey long ago due to its lack of affect. Mum saw this attempt at discipline as abuse. Dad however, took to Simon straight away and thought he would be a steadying influence and supporting his attempts to make Joey behave.

The struggles had terrible knock-on effects for both Mum and Dad as well. Each time Harold agreed with Simon, Mary saw this as going *against* her better judgement. The rows that ensued at this time were hostile and frequent.

Simon tried sending Joey to stand in the corner with his hands on his head when he had a tantrum. Joey just screamed louder and longer. Simon then shouted even louder. Because of Joey's short attention span, each time the child moved or dropped his hands Simon would shout again. Joey would increase on that, and it went on and on. It was an absolute nightmare. Simon thought that by playing Sergeant Major it would scare Joey into submission. No way!

When Joey was bad we threatened him with special school, which we know now was a bad idea. One particular day when we had just had enough, we got Joey dressed and bundled him into the car saying he was going to special school. He screamed and struggled but we put him in the car, took him to an abandoned and dilapidated school building about three miles from where we lived. When we got there we stopped outside and literally threw him out of the car. We were absolutely on the edge, with his hysterical screaming and writhing. Anyone watching would have wondered what on earth was happening. The way I felt that day, I could gladly driven off and left him, but when he calmed down we took him home. This incident did cool Joey off a bit, and he cooperated for a while. Nevertheless we were soon back to the same routines of misbehaviour and inattention.

We were all living in a continuous nightmare. Joey's life was one of horrifying extremes. When he laughed, he laughed hysterically. When he cried, he cried too much. He spoke too loud, ran instead of walking, and was always expending energy on useless movement and noise. He would whistle, hum, burble, sing, tap, waggle his feet, anything just to be doing *something*. He could not control his actions. Like an over-wound spring, we could not gauge what would happen next.

My heart broke to see Joey constantly unsatisfied, not having any friends and always unhappy. I was constantly trying to overcompensate, being extra lenient, extra generous, extra loving. Even though I sometimes felt that I could put my hands round the child's neck and finish him off, my confidence was so weak, that I knew also this was madness, and I was going mad. I couldn't find a positive answer to anything. I didn't know whether or not Simon was in the right. I also knew that the over-compensating did not help. It couldn't because somehow consistency and firm boundary setting with parents pulling together is the only solution.

Sometimes Simon thought I wasn't backing him up in his decisions, and this made him feel an outsider. I couldn't think straight, and was forever searching for reasons for Joey's behaviour. Could it be this, or this? Mum and Dad continued to disagree, and out of all of this, what did I know? I was only the boy's mother! The situation was becoming critical when another nail went into the coffin of our family relationship.

The house we lived in at the time had a coal bunker in a concrete yard at the back. One night Joey was playing on it, climbing up, and dangling off the clothes post immediately next to it. After repeated requests from us to come down, the inevitable happened. Joey fell off the bunker and Simon leapt forward managing to catch Joey by the ankles. Unfortunately this caused Joey to crash down upon the concrete, falling on his arm. Not only had he broken his arm, but his elbow was dislocated. A rush to the Casualty Department that evening revealed that surgery was necessary. We had to leave Joey in the hospital and return to break the news to my parents.

Though not saying it directly, Mum insinuated that Simon was responsible. After all he hated the boy...right? If he hadn't reached out to save Joey, perhaps he would have landed on his feet and come out of it without a scratch. Relations deteriorated even more after this, and reached an all time low. For a long time things were quite strained between us all. Mum did not trust Simon, even though I loved him. Certainly, Simon, due to his background of a strict upbringing and boarding school followed by nine years in the Forces, was perhaps a bit inflexible, but he wasn't a bad or malicious man. Now it seemed that everyone was at each other's throats over one thing or another. Added to this, of course, Joey was still there causing maximum havoc throughout.

Looking back now at those awful times, I wonder why I did not end up in a mental institution. I must be bloody tough underneath. And, why Simon did not just wash his hands of the whole situation I will never know. Each day things were getting worse for Joey at school. He was literally being blamed for any and all disruptions

47

in class, even though he was by no means responsible for beginning it all. Nevertheless his temperament caused him to retaliate inappropriately, and then the teacher would be down on *him* for that.

Though not excusing his behaviour, the school he attended at this time was not addressing his special needs. [We didn't even know what *'special needs'* were then, and the category of person so classified was never mentioned to us.] One day the school were having a concert. Joey was not one of the participants; he was to sit in the rows at the back with the other children. Whilst one child performed, a little girl who was often found to torment Joey gave him a hard shove to make him react. Nothing was said to her, but when Joey pushed her back, the teacher called him out immediately in front of the whole school. Since my mother was in the audience, she saw the whole scenario and was quite rightly furious. But this frequently happened in school to Joey.

The telling off that Joey endured over the years was having a profound effect on him. Unfortunately he just could not differentiate between appropriate and inappropriate behaviour and responses. His impulsiveness mean that he was frequently butting in when the teacher was talking. He wanted an answer, or the teacher's attention NOW. This appeared as extreme rudeness, of course. Joey knew that he was not liked but he could not understand why. It became increasingly difficult to separate incidents when Joey was actually in the wrong from those where he had not been given a fair chance.

In 1994, when Joey was seven, I took him out of school because relations between Joey, the teachers, his peers, and my own relations with the school had deteriorated to such a degree that we could no longer work together. When the old headmaster left and the new headmistress took over, the attitudes within the school had become unhelpful and accusative. Yet, at no time did they ever suggest special needs education, which we now know he should have had from the start, especially after his encephalitis.

I put Joey in another school, without explaining to them the extent of his problems. I suppose I secretly hoped that his behavioural problems were tied up with the old school. By starting a new one the problems might subside. Unfortunately, no. If anything, they got worse. The teachers at the new school were young, inexperienced and simly could not deal with the complex behavioural and emotion problems that Joey was displaying.

Finally, Simon and I went to our family doctor because of my mental state. We poured everything out to him, and he referred us to the local child and adolescent therapy unit. We had one appointment with a psychiatrist before seeing a clinical psychologist for the rest of the sessions. That first appointment did not get very far but I do remember her asking about Joey's hyperactivity. I told her that Joey could concentrate for short periods but only when really interested. Also I informed her of the terrible time he had trying to get off to sleep at night, and the fact he didn't settle till very late with lots of disruption, crashing around the bedroom, coming up and down stairs, asking for drinks of water, bed bouncing, etc. When he eventually did get to sleep he slept right through for five or six hours. Big mistake! Because of this she assumed Joey was not hyperactive, because he could sleep.

[It is thought by some professionals that hyperactive children cannot sleep at all. But, because hyperactivity is just one of a cluster of symptoms which make up ADHD, different children have differing sleep patterns. Some wake many times a night, some will not sleep until the early hours of the morning, some stay up most of the night wandering round the house and getting into scrapes, whereas some sleep six to eight hours once they eventually get down to it. Also, children with ADD (without hyperactivity) sometimes sleep too much.]

The whole series of appointments that followed with the clinical psychologist, therefore, were based on the assumption that Joey was not hyperactive. It then followed that another reason for his inexplicable behaviour had to be found. On subsequent appointments the family situation was explored. We discussed the disagreements between family members as to the correct way to be parents to Joey. It came out loud and clear that Mary was isolated in her opinions about the way we were trying to bring Joey up. Since Harold and Simon agreed that more discipline was called for and I felt in the middle, whatever decisions I made would upset someone. My wavering wasn't giving Joey a clear indication of what was expected of him. It was decided, much to Mary's disgust, that Simon and I only, should set guidelines of what was expected and stick to them no matter what. This did help slightly because the psychologist gave me back some confidence to make decisions regarding Joey. At least she seemed to have confidence in my ability.

In making decisions, Simon and I stuck together as much as possible. I still thought that Simon occasionally went over the top with his discipline or punishment. I abided by Simon's decisions however, and then, later on, would take up with him any unfairness I thought he had shown. This device was to lessen Joey's chances of playing us off against each other as he had grown rather adept at doing. Nevertheless I felt guilty for letting Simon have the last word so often, however much it eased the pressure.

Another method we tried was a system of rewards, such as ignoring bad behaviour and rewarding good. This emphatically did not work. The trouble with this is that any parent does this sort of thing instinctively anyway, as it seems the most positive way of supporting a child's good behaviour. I explained to the psychologist that we had already tried this strategy, but we would try it again. It really was a dead loss. Although Joey responded at first for a reward, once he got the hang of it, he wanted bigger and bigger rewards. He would only agree to cooperate for two rewards, then three. Then three plus ten pence, and so on. Since this set of attempts did not work, we abandoned that strategy.

In our explorations it became apparent to the psychologist how bright Joey really is, and therefore it was difficult for her to perceive how such a clever boy could have severe behavioural and temperamental problems. He was well behaved at these sessions because everything was novel and he was the center of attention. The extent of his difficulties did not show up and the amount of strife ensuing in the family due them did not emerge.

Diary
We all have the therapy sessions next week again. God, these appointments are really getting me down. We go along and talk about what is happening, but Joey is perfect for those 40 minutes or so, and it is really difficult to get across the difficulties. When we leave, he behaves like an animal let loose. It therefore appears that Joey is just boisterous and we are incompetent parents. Mary is being so stubborn. She has this way of making me feel that I am the one with the problem, not Joey. But I know that this way of living is not right and I know that Joey is ill. He is so restless and hyperactive, like a car engine which is racing. I am so frightened.

We went to family therapy sessions at intervals, but in September of 1994 we were discharged as nothing could be done for us. We had been trying to manage Joey's neurological condition with psychological methods. We were told that Joey had no emotional disturbances which could account for his behaviour. Therefore these were basically put down to Joey's high intelligence making him bored at school. The boredom was thought to be making him disruptive, in combination with the lack of consistent boundary setting by us. The solution was thought to be slight adjustments by ourselves and extra homework given by the school. In the psychologists' opinion these slight adaptations by ourselves would wipe out five years plus of home and school problems and all the knock-on effects that had been caused in the family. Following is the final report by the psychologist.

Counselling and therapy service, Children and adolescents, September 1994

Dear Dr. A., Re: Joey Miller (28.2.87)

Following a referral from Dr. B, consultant in child and adolescent psychiatry, Joey was seen with his mother by our family therapy team on three occasions, one of which included his maternal grandparents. We have explored the need for consistent boundary setting for Joey which we feel is especially important as he is such an intelligent little boy. We now feel that Mrs. Miller and her new husband are uniting in their approach to the issue and Joey's behaviour has improved considerably. Whilst there remain some situations where his behaviour is difficult we feel that the family know the way to handle these effectively. We have agreed no more appointments are required but should this change within the next six months the family can arrange another by contacting us directly.

Yours sincerely, A.C., Senior Clinical Practitioner

Simon and I had been married in August. Joey was seven and a half at the time, and I was also expecting a baby due in January, 1995. Meanwhile at school, things were not improving. Joey's inability to cope was ongoing, and everyone was becoming fed up with him just as previously. I knew he was troublesome, but I also knew he was not always treated fairly. He was in trouble every day. His school work was far behind the others despite his high intelligence. The frustration was overwhelming, and the problem never ending. I knew Joey was bright as his teachers did, and he himself knew it too, yet he was still failing miserably.

Joey started to complain that no one would listen to him. He said that teachers always took other children's side. That is when his frustrations exploded with devastating consequences for himself and others around him. When he had a particularly bad day at school, he would come home and take it out on us. His own anger and frustration at how he was treated by others put him under unsustainable pressure on top of his other outstanding problems of inattention and hyperactivity. His blind rages were not only frightening for us but also dangerous for him as he could injure himself badly when he crashed about or banged his head against the wall.

He believed that the teachers hated him. There were numerous incidents of scapegoating going on, and the poor child's self image was as a 'hate object'. He began showing sure signs of depression and defeat. Paradoxically however, the lower his morale sunk the higher his activity level rose. He was like an over-wound spring, whizzing here, there and everywhere in utter confusion. School was now a hell on earth for him. When I collected him in the afternoon to bring him home, as the children poured out of class I would be greeted with "Joey's done this," "Joey's done that" or "Teacher is keeping Joey in".....again! This got so bad for me that I began dropping Joey off at Mum's in the morning, and she would take him back and forth to school.

It was a truly horrible feeling to have a young teacher in her twenties, with no children of her own, and with no knowledge of you or your situation, to be asking you if you realised that your child has low self esteem, is rude and aggressive, constantly butts in on conversations, gets up and walks about the class. Of course we knew! Our only thoughts could be, "Yeah, so what? What do you think we can do about it?"

I had been searching for an answer for over 6 years by this time. The school knew this. It wasn't as if we had just washed our hands of Joey and let him get on with it. We had tried every avenue we knew and consulted the health professionals, all in a desperate attempt to get help for him. No mention had ever been made of special needs assistance at either of the schools he had attended. If I had only known then what I know now, I would have pushed for the extra help long ago. I could not push for something I did not know existed.

The situation was really impossible. I had thought the previous school was bad, but this one....

Joey had been surrounded by negative responses since being eighteen months old. He had endured the frustration and anger at home and our disagreements over the situation. He had few friends and suffered the isolation of that alongside the day in and day out agony of school. He was not invited to birthday parties, never picked to be in the school play, was always tutted and blamed even when he was not at fault. The negative reinforcement of teachers who disliked him and were quick to scold and punish was such a heavy burden for these young shoulders. He was extremely depressed and at seven years old was threatening suicide.

He called himself 'dumb' and 'worthless', he took no pride in his appearance, and looked as if he had been pulled through a hedge backwards. When we tried to straighten his clothes or tidy him up, help was refused. He punished himself, and really appeared to think it wasn't worth the effort. My heart broke for him, because I wanted to take his pain away but couldn't.

The examples of his scapegoating are too numerous to relate, though a few of these may be helpful to other parents going through this special type of hell.

One day when the teacher was having a problem with him, the class of seven year olds was asked to vote whether or not to evict Joey from the classroom. They voted him out. He went out into the corridor for the rest of the day. Even I find it hard to imagine what that would do to a child who already has the most fragile grip on life. If I had been stronger at the time I would have had the teacher up before the authorities. But I was terribly confused and worn out, helpless and growing bigger and more vulnerable by the day with my pregnancy.

Another day when Mum had taken Joey into school, she was waiting for him outside of the toilets prior to seeing him into the classroom. Imagine her surprise when she got into class with Joey, to hear another little boy telling the teacher that Joey had just hit him (when he hadn't even arrived yet!) This certainly gave us an insight into what was actually going on at the school. True, Joey was challenging, but other mothers frequently approached me to relate episodes when Joey had got the blame and been punished for things for which he had not been at fault.

Mum went across to watch Joey on one of the school sports days when I was ill. When all the children came out onto the field, Joey was escorted back inside, and banned from playing for the apparent throwing of a shoe. What had actually happened was that Joey was *returning* the shoe that had been thrown at him by another child. Child No. 1 played while Joey was punished.

Once Joey locked himself in the toilet and stuck his head down the bowl. Another time he cut his fringe off right at the roots and had no fringe at all for months. He was often found shouting and screaming at teachers. Apart from the fact of his scapegoating, he had to live each day with the inability to concentrate on a task, aware that no one liked him, and with the frustration that everyone seemed to know what they were doing when he did not.

Looking back, it was so unfair, and writing this I have tears running down my face. Firstly I cry because of the anger I feel at the actions and inactions of that school, but also because of my inability at the time to do anything to help my son. I let them get away with it and I will never forgive myself for not doing more. The years had worn me down, and I was not the same person I had been, nor have become again in recent years.

After our marriage, Simon and I decided to take a holiday with Joey, as a sort of a honeymoon, but it turned out to be the holiday from hell. Joey was in a terrible state, depressed, angry with us and the world. Simon was on the defensive the whole time because of my Mum and I was a nervous wreck. Joey banged his head up against the walls, threw things or tried to harm himself by gouging his forearms with his fingernails. Sometimes he picked up a heavy toy and banged it against his head or body in temper. We did try to contain him as much as possible, but it was maniacal the way he argued, answered back over every matter and was so oppositional. He couldn't remember things, and his mind was in utter confusion. He was so bad at following instructions that he would almost do the opposite of what was being asked of him. It was as if his brain worked backwards.

Off we went to Blackpool, me four and a half months pregnant with sciatica sending severe shooting pains down my leg. From the moment we started it was one long argument. Joey was on top form of awkwardness the whole time and kept egging Simon on with his cheekiness, which I had to listen to all day. Because Joey was so high, upset and whinging the whole time, we did try to buy him off by giving him more and more money to put in the slot machines. Not only did it not satisfy him, but when we finally called it quits, Joey threw the most horrific tantrum in a public place. He seemed to want to spoil things at every opportunity and finally we got so fed up that we took photos each time he burst into tears. We came back with some priceless ones of Joey in various states of agitation just to prove to his Grandma what he was like on holiday.

One day was particularly horrific and I didn't feel at all well. Simon was edgy because of the gathering stress, and by lunch time I was ready to get on a train and leave them to it. Joey got a real telling off along the Golden Mile while astonished holidaymakers looked on. That evening we all sat in stony silence throughout our meal, Joey clearing his throat and blinking his eyes the whole time.

Often sufferers of neurological conditions have tics like Joey. His are both vocal and facial and they first began to show up at about the age of five, when the real problems at school had also emerged. Mum put the tics down to nerves, in other words, the stress we putting him under. His tics went in phases and began with clearing his throat repeatedly. this would become worse when he was confused or especially hyperactive. He also went through a phase of wrinkling his nose like a rabbit, then a period of blinking his eyes and scrunching up his face. We tried not to draw attention to the tics to avoid making them worse. The blinking lasted for a while and then he moved onto rolling his eyeballs upwards under his eye lids. All of these mannerisms were involuntary and he really couldn't control them. Currently he sniffs incessantly, which doesn't look so bad, but is really irritating to hear.

On one morning of our holiday we visited the zoo. After returning to the hotel, we sat Joey down and asked him to write the names of twenty animals he had seen that day. First he refused, then after what seemed an eternity of asking, pleading, bribing and shouting at him, we finally got him sitting in one place with a pad of paper and pen. After trying to stall us by making excuses and asking for drinks, then some screaming, he finally wrote "one lion and nineteen penguins." He thought this was a perfectly logical answer, and in some ways, of course, it was quite a clever reply. But the truth was that he couldn't remember twenty different animals, and being Joey, he would rather get himself into trouble than admit his lack of memory.

Anyway, Blackpool was a total disaster and we came back vowing "never again".

7

Heading towards a nervous breakdown

Diary
I have been drinking again, my hands are shaking and I can hardly breathe. I have had another big row with Mum. Can't she see what is happening? She only seems to feel for him but WHAT ABOUT ME? Does anyone think about me? This week has seen Joey reduce me to tears every day. I am on the verge of tears at all

times now anyway though, so it doesn't take much to start me off.

After our holiday, the school term started again, and so did our nightmare. Joey was always being kept behind after school to account for his misdemeanours. After setting off from home at about ten past three to pick him at half past, I had to wait until all the kids came out of the classroom and been taken away by their mums. At about twenty to four the teacher addressed Joey about such and such an incident, and then I had to go into the classroom or to the headmistress's office, to see what crimes he had committed that day. This took time, and it got so that I was not getting home until well after four. Looking back now, I realise all of this was absurd. I was about six to seven months pregnant by this time, stressed to the extreme and extremely vulnerable. I felt as if the school were taking it out on me, and not even trying to understand Joey.

Most of the time Joey did not know why he was in trouble. It is not difficult to understand how a comment or jibe from a classmate, which would bounce off any child with a normal temperament, instantly sent him rocketing into orbit. Because he was always on the defensive, after repeated bullying and attacks on him, he was not good at just reacting verbally; his response was to lash out physically. This could not be tolerated in school of course. But this was the only way that Joey knew to try and fend off the blame. And his memory was so bad that he forgot what he had actually done in the first place.

Diary
My life recently has been one long round of hassle and misery. I am in at the school every day because Joey is causing havoc, but at the same time he is extremely depressed because of the situation. I have asked for the educational psychologist in to assess Joey, but

the headmistress says he is not bad enough. Why are they making my life such a misery then by hauling me in every night? I cannot do anything to change Joey, so what is accomplished by recounting every little thing to me? Some of the things I am brought in for are so trivial. If a normal child had done these things, nothing would be said, but because Joey is difficult to start with, everything is compounded and reported. Mum is on my back too because of it all. She wants me to cause trouble at the education department about the situation but I am so tired, so, so tired. The fight has been knocked out of me over the last seven years....

My emotions were on a roller coaster when these things happened. I wanted to reach in and get through to his heart and head and take the pain away. At the same time his negative and aggressive behaviour and his refusal to accept help was also making my own life a misery. With the teachers on at him all day and the torment again from us at home, he was a child separated from us by an impenetrable barrier. We simply could not reach him.

His physical appearance was a subtle but ongoing torture to us all. He would have one sock on, one sock off, shoe laces untied, shirt hanging out and jumper back to front. This is when he began the day; it may seem to other parents today that all of their children in school uniforms or not, look like this by the end of the day. But Joey could not figure out how dressing himself worked and yet he did not want help. He would virtually always put his top on back to front, with the label sticking out under his chin. He did it so often that I really thought he was doing it out of devilment but he wasn't. He had no coordination and could not get the hang of putting his shoes on the right feet, and typing shoe laces! He wore shoes with Velcro fastening till he was seven and a half.

When I sent him straight to bed at night because I had just had enough, I would find him in the morning with his pyjamas over his daytime clothes. When I tried to explain to him why this wasn't the thing to do, he could not understand that what he was doing was wrong. It was not a life and death mistake admittedly, but time was moving on and Joey should have been able to dress and undress himself by this age. Even now at eleven years old he cannot understand how you put on night clothes to go to bed, and start again next morning with fresh daytime clothes. Without supervision of the closest sort he would just wear the same clothes week in, week out.

He also forgot to put pants on, or on sports days at school he would come home with his uniform on top of his P.E. kit. It wasn't worth the hassle for him to try to undress, put his kit away in his bag, and dress in his uniform again: the easiest way for him was to put layer over layer.

Diary
What have I been put on this earth for? I feel just like a punch-bag. Everyone has a piece of me, and I have been lost along the way. Joey's difficulties are so severe now that I absolutely despair. My head hurts, my chest is tight, and I have difficulty breathing. I have frequent palpitations, my hands shake and this lump in my throat feels like it is getting bigger. Some days I feel like killing myself, I really do, but what would happen to the baby I am carrying?

The pregnancy is getting me down, and I am scared that this baby might be like Joey. What if he or she has the same temperament? What if the baby won't settle at night, just like him? My own sleep is poor anyway. How will I cope with even less sleep. I feel like I am not living. I am just existing in a nightmare. Everyday is a mixture of aggravation, stress, sadness and despondency. It is a swirling and vicious circle with no escape, no options and no hope.

In 1995, when Joey was eight, I gave birth to our daughter Emily, whose birth could not have been more different from Joey's. It was a text book delivery with no pain relief, no stitches and no complications. But on the day I went into labour, I had been called into the headmistress at Joey's school to listen to her complaints through my contractions. Obviously the whole situation was intolerable, and Simon and I decided, after the delivery, to contact the family therapy unit again. But, if one could even have said that we were hopeful of help, we were doomed to disappointment. We had to continue to wonder about what these so-called professionals actually do for their money? We came away again without being any further on; their findings follow, but I had to then surmise that they attended a different session to our own.

"Joey was seen again on 20.4.95 along with his mother, stepfather and new sister, at his mother's request. During the interview Joey appeared to be well behaved and settled, and said he felt very happy with the situation at home. The parents reported that mother and stepfather continued to maintain clear and appropriate boundaries, and everyone felt the situation at home was much improved.

Further questioning around the situation suggested that Joey's difficult behaviour in school might be associated with boredom rather than any underlying management problem or any unresolved traumatic issue for Joey himself. No further family sessions were set up but it was suggested that the issue of Joey's ability should be therefore discussed at school."

Diary
Today, I pulled up outside the house to find about two miles of cassette tape wrapped around the satellite dish, and all round the telephone wires. I asked Joey if he had a cassette tape today, and he replied with an emphatic no. I went next door to borrow our neighbour's ladder in order to get the tape down. "He's a little tinker isn't he?" said the neighbour.
"What?" I asked.

He explained that he knew the cassette tape Joey had yesterday would come to grief, as he had seen him unravelling it in the wind and knew it would end up somewhere it shouldn't.

When faced with it, Joey eventually admits he did steal one of my tapes yesterday and then went on to protest that I had asked him about today, not yesterday. I realised I was just wasting my time.

We were back to square one then. It was arranged for the school nurse to come in to test Joey's hearing, just in case this had something to do with his problematic behaviour. Both his ears and eyes were tested, and both proved perfect. What now? I was still returning to the health visitor at times, trying to get help. Years had passed since I first contacted her and she was getting quite sick of me by now. I was desperate however, and felt myself heading for a nervous breakdown on the fast track. As I was trying to explain what Joey's behaviour was like I could see that she simply could not or would not understand.

I remember her asking me "Does he read books?" God, I wished! He couldn't sit in one place long enough. She had not the faintest idea of what I was trying to tell her; relations between the two of us were getting bad because I was frustrated with her lack of an answer but also angry that someone working in a profession which specialised in child health was so ignorant about this uncontrollable level of activity of Joey's. She could not help me but I would not drop it. Impasse. I feared for Joey's safety and my sanity. The way things were going, murder was on the menu. And though I realised that it was totally irrational, I threatened to dump him on the Social Services. Still nothing happened and no one could help.

Diary
Mum rang up this morning in a terrible state. I had dropped Joey
off at her house for her to take him into school, and he had been
playing with some tools in the outhouse before she could get him
into the car. When she got back home after dropping him off, she
noticed that the Stanley knife was missing, and though she wasn't
sure, her suspicions were roused. She dashed back to the school and
sure enough, he had sneaked the thing into school. There it was
in his coat pocket. God, I dread to think what could have
happened.....his actions are so totally incomprehensible.

School broke up for the summer and although the
hassle I was getting from the headmistress would cease
for a few months, Joey would be there all day and every
day, and I dreaded it. I was drained of all energy and did
not want to get up each morning. Joey's school report
arrived and it was a catalogue of failure. There were
comments in the report such as "lacks concentration"
and "doesn't take into account the feelings and needs of
others." It was if by putting it in writing to me — all
those things about Joey which I knew already and was
constantly being chastised for at the school — there was
some idea that I could sternly talk with him, and turn
him into a model pupil?

After reading the school report a few times and
having a damn good cry (not for the first time) I flew
down to the health visitor's office again to plead with
her for help. I took the report with the problematic
behaviour comments underlined. Perhaps she would
believe me now? She was still at a loss as to what to
suggest. I cried and even screamed at her....surely there
was SOMEONE in Yorkshire who could help us? She
could think of no one. I asked her to refer me back to
the paediatrician who had looked after Joey when he
had encephalitis, but she said this would be
inappropriate. Alternatively she offered to refer me to
the school doctor, to see if he might have any

suggestions. I received an appointment but it was not to be until August. In the meantime something happened.

8

The Breakthrough

This was the summer of 1995. Joey was eight and a half years, and baby Emily was six and a half months old. I went to see the doctor and told her all that was happening. I told her that whenever I put Emily down for naps or to sleep at night, Joey would invariably wake her with his crashing about. Emily would then be grumpy too, Joey would be in trouble, and Simon and I were either arguing or I was in tears. My alcohol consumption increased in the attempt to get some sort of relaxation. The whole household was out of control, what with crying and nappies and teething, and arguing. I lived with a constant headache and gripping pains in my chest.

The doctor said, "I think you need a holiday." Absolutely not, no thank you, not after the last one....that's for sure. She sent me away with no help, no medication, no counselling, nothing. I was alone in my misery and alone with my one big problem. That problem called Joey.

One morning I was listening to Talk Radio and tuned into Anna Raeburn's 'agony hour'. The program often consoled me, perhaps because there were other people out there with problems, different to mine, admittedly, but with problems nevertheless. It seemed to lift me out of myself to listen. The show consisted of an hour on a specific subject, after which she would take phone calls from listeners.

On this particular day she was interviewing a guest about *problem children*. My ears pricked up, and as the interview continued, tingles began running up and down my spine, and goose bumps came up on my arms. The interviewee was describing my Joey!

They talked about a neurological condition they were calling *Attention Deficit Hyperactivity Disorder*, or ADHD for short. The symptoms attributed to this condition were mainly inattentiveness, hyperactivity, impulsivity and insatiability. The more I listened, the more I was engrossed. If left untreated, the condition worsens and there are all of the knock-on effects which I recognised: disruptiveness at school, aggressive behaviour, and low self esteem. I was dumbfounded to hear that a drug was available which had proven positive effects on sufferers, often dramatic, but since ADHD was not well or widely recognised in Britain, it was not easy to get the medication at that time. Then, to my utter amazement, listeners began to call in and describe their children. The same problems that we had been facing for so long were recounted again and again.

Just like us, the callers had consulted numerous professionals in an attempt to get help for their children. I just could not believe it because every caller that came on could have been me speaking. One parent after another described the hell that we were going through. By the end of the program I was shaking with anger and crying my eyes out. The burst of emotion experienced left me numb. Could it possibly be that I was not going mad after all? Everything seemed surreal and I was left wondering if I had just dreamed the last hour. I pinched myself hard to ensure I was awake. The program had passed so quickly so I tried to recall everything that was said. I then sat staring at the radio for what seemed ages, but was probably only minutes. My mind was working overtime as the last seven or eight years flashed up before my eyes. Finally I calmly got out the whisky and had a large drink. Then I had another, my mind buzzing all the time. I cried a bit more, screamed at the walls, had *another* drink then waited for Simon to come home.

If this condition was real, why had we been fobbed off, passed from pillar to post all these years? Why had Joey's condition not been taken seriously? The psychiatrist and psychologist had both worked on the premise that it was external circumstances that caused Joey's problems and that parental techniques or lack of them had been to blame for Joey's problems. Why wasn't the condition more widely known about, recognised, or even accepted as real? Why had ADHD never even been mentioned by the professional educators and doctors as well as the specialists? This radio programme was the first in which I had ever heard the term — *Attention Deficit Hyperactivity Disorder*. The name was not easy, but forgetting it now was impossible.

I was relieved because for the first time in years I could see a light — a tiny light, yes, but a light nonetheless, at the end of a very long tunnel. But also I felt angry too. Very angry. Why had we suffered so long, especially Joey? My mood changed from melancholy to near elation.....could we now move forward with our lives?

What I heard on this program convinced me that this condition was what afflicted Joey. The symptoms and the behaviours were exactly the same ones as he had displayed over the years. Hyperactivity as toddler, turning into disruptiveness at school. Lack of concentration or attention leading to frustration and aggressiveness. Expulsion from school and so on. Everything fitted exactly. The man interviewed by

67

Anna Raeburn was representing the National ADHD Family Support Group, whose address I had taken down. I wrote asking for their literature the same afternoon. Ironically, that very same week I saw an article by Dr. Chris Steel in *T.V. Quick*, the television magazine which was also about ADHD. It listed all the symptoms, and on reading this, I was even more sure that Joey was a sufferer.

After reading the leaflets which arrived from the support group a few days later I knew that it was true: Joey was suffering from ADHD. Fate was lending us a hand. If only this had happened years earlier....

ADHD is a neurological condition in which the sufferer has a deficiency of certain brain chemicals, and the problems it presents stem from the underfunctioning of those areas of the brain which put the brakes on unwise behaviour — the frontal lobes. It is as if sufferers have no sense of inhibition. The condition is hereditary and is thought to affect about one in twenty school age children.[ADHD leaflet, text by Dr. Christopher Green]

There we were, thinking we were the worst parents in the whole world, and the only ones with a child like this. With a condition reportedly so common, psychiatrists and psychologists had to be seeing children like this quite frequently and then denying them proper help. Where were their so-called scientific methods that could not pick up on many common behavioural problems and at least suspect there could be a biological base. Experts are supposed to be clever, and of course, they are obliged to keep up on their professional literature. At least, they should *know* about it.

After digesting the literature from the support group, I was convinced that I had to take this further. I now knew that Joey had ADHD and my next move was to get him to someone who recognised the condition and could actually help us. I rang the support group and spoke to a friendly woman. I described our family history, and explained how we had tried to explore every avenue in the attempt to get help for Joey. Our story was all too familiar.

She told me that ADHD was only just becoming recognised in this country although the Americans and the Australians had been treating the disorder for years with great success. Finding anyone here with the expertise was and remains very difficult. Families are still trailing from one specialist to another and not only being denied help but also being made to feel that their children's problems are their own fault.

She gave me the name of a consultant at St James Hospital in Leeds, less than eight miles from where I lived. Our appointment with the school doctor was coming up shortly so I decided to ask him to refer us to this same specialist at St. James'. Meanwhile I wrote to the health visitor explaining what I had discovered, and saying that I was going to ask for a referral. She wasn't impressed because she hadn't heard or read about this condition, and yet here was someone who works with children on a daily basis. Subsequently I was to learn that the great majority of professionals who work with our children — health visitors, social workers, teachers, paediatricians, family doctors, psychologists and psychiatrists are on the whole uninformed about the disorder, and many also have a strong resistence to educating themselves about it as well.

As an educational measure, my first foray but certainly not my last, I took the support group material down to her office. This provided her with the list of diagnostic criteria, the signs and symptoms to look out for, a description of what caused the disorder, etc. Her immediate reaction to me was to ask a question: "Could Joey be dyslexic?" She just wasn't listening or taking in

69

the material. She was clutching at straws related to what she already knew. Reflecting on this experience, I realised that she like many other professionals do not much care for the idea of parents taking a pro-active approach and trying to find their own solutions to problems. I told her that I would have my referral to St. James and that I would come back at a later date to prove to her that I was right and not imagining all the problems we had endured.

On reading *Understanding ADHD*, by Dr. Christopher Green, a book which I had been advised to buy, a hundred light bulbs lit up in my head. There was not one thing in it, that did not apply to Joey. I could also begin to identify the symptoms and behaviours in Joey's father too and even in myself to some extent, in that it was made clear that this was a hereditary medical condition. The book included descriptions of how family relations are marred, and the attendant educational underachievement. Simon and I pored over the book so much that it was looseleaved very quickly. Joey's grandparents were not convinced at first. It has taken Dad quite a time to understand and accept that the behaviours are caused by neurological disturbance and not by naughtiness. After reading the book cover to cover, Mum soon agreed.

Mum came along to the interview with the school doctor and ourselves to give moral support. This time we were determined that we wouldn't be sent away without help. With Dr. Green's book we had documentary evidence that there was an affliction which was recognised in other countries as a legitimate neurological condition, and we were also sure that this was at the root of Joey's problems. To make it easy for the school doctor, we gave him the name of the consultant that we needed to see, and really left him with no alternative but to go along with our wishes. I suppose he had expected us to go in all ears to hear what he could suggest. Instead we told him what we wanted, what we expected from him, and that we would not leave that day without the referral. His initial reply was that he could not refer us because he worked for the Wakefield Health Authority and we wanted to see a doctor in the Leeds area. Well, I will spare you how I responded to that!

He then offered to give our case to our family doctor, asking him to refer us. This was accepted as the best way forward. Our own doctor had not heard of ADHD before either, but he nevertheless seemed interested in the literature I took in with me. He promised to read it, and that made a refreshing change. Once again, of course, we would be building up our confidence in order to see a new specialist, and have to go through the whole sorry story again. This time however I felt a glimmer of hope. If the specialist knew about ADHD and was treating it, surely he would recognise Joey as a typical example. I waited for my appointment to come through....and waited and waited.

I rang the hospital to find out why I had not received the appointment for Joey, to be told that they had received no referral from my doctor and had never even heard of Joey Miller. I was like a volcano by this point. I rang my local health centre and asked the receptionist to get the health visitor on the phone NOW!

I hung on the end of the phone for what seemed like an eternity, all the time fuming and going over in my head what I was going to say. I convinced myself that as soon as she knew it was me she would not come to the phone. I was transferred from one department to another, until a voice came at the other end: "Mrs. Miller?"

I am ashamed to say I let rip. I screamed at her that I was not impressed after coming this far to be

71

continually hampered in my efforts to get help for our family, help to which we were entitled. Was there some conspiracy going on? She quickly went to get the referral notes from my doctor's files, and assured me that she would get the letter off the same day. Imagine my surprise when about an hour later I had a call from the specialist's secretary at St. James. Miraculously Joey's referral had turned up. *Great thing these fax machines!*

My appointment for Joey came through the post and it was for three weeks time. I was over the moon! The date would be 6 October, 1995.

9

6th October 1995

St. James' is a large teaching hospital featured in the television show Jimmys. The Specialist's clinic is located in a separate building in the grounds of the main hospital. The time of our appointment finally arrived and is difficult to put into words the emotions I experienced that day. I was excited, fearful, hopeful, frightened and my thoughts veered from positive to negative to positive again. By this time I had pored over all the information and believed I knew a lot about ADHD. I also knew that the condition could be treated medically with dramatic results for some sufferers. Joey was getting older, his childhood had been all but lost, and I had to go into this thing wholeheartedly in order to try and make up for lost time. And apart from the medication, I wanted affirmation that I had been right all along and that Joey did have an impairment, he was not a bad boy, and that we were not bad parents.

On the 6th of October we went as a family group, Simon, my Mum, Joey and I, hoping against hope that the specialist would help us. I looked and felt a complete wreck, and much more akin to a 50 year old than my actual 35 years. I was pale, haggard, drained and exhausted, and everyone could see it. Joey was in his own world and very depressed.

Our first shock was in arriving in the waiting room of the clinic and finding a number of "Joeys" crashing around, screaming, jumping off things and generally causing chaos. All we could hear was "No Carl!" or "Stop it Craig!" It was funny really, to see how similar many of these children were, some with blonde or mousy coloured hair and blue eyes just like Joey. They all had that certain crazed look in their eyes, a bit like Jack Nicholson on an off day.

The specialist called us in. He was a quiet, rotund little man, a lot younger than I had expected. I am sure he could tell just by looking at us just how desperate we all were. We recounted to him the terrible time we had been living through over the past seven years. I told him that I was tired, tired of fighting with health visitors, tired of having to justify myself to teachers, fed up of having other people look at me as a bad parent because I couldn't control my child. He took Joey's medical history, gave him a physical examination and read through the school reports, all while listening to me pouring my heart out to him. We explained how we had seen several so-called specialists none of whom had offered any real help, how bad the situation had been at the last two schools and how we were putting Joey in a new school right now, the third he had been to in his short school career. The doctor could see how ragged I was and could also see the very depressed little boy sitting there.

He then explained about a medication which had been found to have a very beneficial effect on children like Joey. It is called Ritalin (or Methylphenidate), and he was prepared to start Joey on just half a tablet to start off with, and he was prepared to do that right then. He took Joey into the ante room and gave him the small dose immediately.

I burst into tears. Mum burst into tears and I just remember saying out loud "Thank God, Thank God, Thank God" over and over again. Mum cried, not from frustration and distress this time, but from sheer relief and a hope for the future for this poor little boy who had lost out on his childhood. We were all overcome with the feeling that after all these years of fighting to get help, this moment was the turning point. The specialist looked at the condition from a medical point of view, not a psychological one, and he had no doubts as to the authenticity of every word we said. He didn't condemn us, accuse us, or make us feel that we were in the wrong. Not only did he listen to us, he heard what we were saying to him, and had been saying to many others over the years. He agreed with us that Joey did have an attention deficit. There was a malfunction in Joey's head.

We left St. James' elated. On the way back from the hospital the atmosphere in the car was very calm. I glanced through my driver's mirror to look at Joey and he was asleep, in the middle of the afternoon! When we got home the atmosphere in the house was like nothing I had known before. Joey smiled, walked instead of crashing about, and even got out some pencils and paper to draw a picture. Joey was calm. That night was the first night that we had not been at each other's throats. Later we watched the television for a half hour....an unknown phenomenon. For the first time in years my heart was not racing twenty to the dozen. I felt reasonably calm, but at the same time astonished at the difference in Joey in such a brief period of time.

Let me hasten to add, however, that this was not the end of the long road for us. It was just the beginning.

Diary
Joey has been on Ritalin for a week now and appears to be doing very well on it. He is much calmer and less restless, although it is difficult to put my finger on exactly what is different about him. His personality is exactly the same but he is less wound up somehow. He is not sedated in any way, but then again he is not crashing about so much. We have still had one or two blow ups, but not to the same extent. The School teachers have already noticed the change in his handwriting, because it is neat now that he is taking medication. And most definitely, his concentration span has lengthened.

Some weeks on.

Diary
Joey is going to his Dad's for four days. Hurrah! It may sound cruel but any parent of a challenging child will recognise the enormous sigh of relief one feels when the family has a break from a child like this. Joey has definitely been doing better recently, but every day is still sheer hard work. Simon and I haven't had such a long break from Joey for ages, not since Bill took him last time. At least Joey goes to Bill's at the weekends on normal weeks too. On particularly bad weeks these weekends enable us to recharge batteries, so to speak. Since Bill is going to take Joey for a little holiday, this will give Simon, Emily and I are going to have a few days away together as well, a chance to spend time as a normal family for once.

Then days later.

Diary
Joey came down the stairs this morning in one of his sulks. How
can someone get out of bed in the morning in such a surly mood?
"Hiya" says Simon.
No answer.
"Hiya" Simon repeats.
"I said hiya" retorts Joey.
Oh God, here we go again. It is going to be one of those days. Some
days start with a quarrel, and run into one long and never-ending
argument. Today looks like one of them. By afternoon we feel like
we have done ten rounds with Frank Bruno!

10

Attention Deficit Hyperactivity Disorder

When Joey had begun in the new school in September, I had gone straight to the headmistress and admitted to her that Joey had behavioural problems and that this was the third school he had attended. Since Joey had been at the new school for about three weeks before the specialist appointment came through, his new headmistress and teacher had seen and experienced Joey prior to any diagnosis and treatment.

A major plus about the new school was the accommodation it made for special needs children. The headmistress who was also the special needs coordinator, asked me if I thought it would be beneficial to bring the 'statementing procedure' in for Joey? Since I had never heard of it before, I didn't, of course, know what it was.

A school can make special provision for children with special educational needs. For example, a child may need extra tuition, special equipment or other accommodations in school to help him/her with their education.

I had first to wonder why the other two schools had offered nothing of the sort, but then we agreed that statementing would be beneficial, and she put the whole process in motion. She did warn me that it could be some months before any specific help for Joey was forthcoming, but the school was applying for an assistant to come and work with him on a one to one basis for as many hours as possible. Ideally the assistant would be full time, since the child benefits so much from this steady contact. And also the classroom teacher is freed to concentrate on the remainder of the class without unnecessary disruption.

Meantime, Joey had started on his medication, first twice and then three times a day. The change in him was unbelievable. He was calmer, happier, and it was if some of the unnecessary external distractions were eliminated from his hearing. His handwriting improved tremendously, and his class teacher was astonished; she said that Joey's writing was like the work of a new person altogether.

At home the whole atmosphere was calmer but this would not be described as normal. Joey was still highly strung, tempermental and still could blow up at the slightest thing. But to us there was improvement. No doubt about it.

To go forward on the two fronts: home and school, was our aim. Though the difference was obvious to the school, Joey's classwork improved, and the teachers were pleased, he still had a big problem with his explosive personality. The habits of his lifetime behaviours could not be remedied overnight. The

77

Headmistress decided to bring in the educational psychologist to work with Joey to attempt to pinpoint the biggest problem areas. Perhaps it would have been simpler to pinpoint the areas which were not a problem: there were fewer of those!

Diary
Joey is on an even keel at the moment and we are starting to get the odd flash of brilliance from him. He is thinking more clearly for sure. Our acceptance of him definitely helps. We now know that Joey does have a condition but it is really difficult trying to convince other people that a biological condition can cause such behavioural problems.

There have been some stories in the press recently with headlines such as "It's just another name for naughty children" or "It's a load of codswallop", which is really insulting, coming as it does from the pens of ignorant people. There is nothing so vile as the uninformed non-sufferer lecturing to the educated!

Meantime I had written to the Education Authority asking them to do a statutory assessment for special needs assistance. When a parent requests this, there is the imperative of having to move quickly. The statementing procedure usually takes about six months so it was not something which was going to come into operation immediately. But with the help of the school's Head, I felt confident enough again to start fighting for my own son.

We continued to have a few ups and downs with Joey at school. For example, he could still be aggressive with the other children and got into a number of fights. I did have to keep going in to the school at first to monitor the situation with the staff. But their attitudes were a breath of fresh air and completely different from the other two schools. They took a positive approach to sorting out problems, they were not confrontational, accusative, and generally they were very sympathetic to what we had gone through and were still going through. They bent over backwards to help Joey. I never once had the impression that they hated them, rather they seemed to be genuinely fond of him. At least they cared about his welfare and due to this, he seemed to improve. We knew he had a lot of catching up to do, and that he would never really be on a par with the other children of his own age, but at least we were making headway and going in the right direct.

The improvements I observed at home were in everyday things such as Joey dressing himself. Whereas before the jumper would be on backwards every time, now he might just get it right some of the time. Once I even saw him looking at the label inside of the neck first to see which way it had to go. To me this was a major breakthrough because he was thinking prior to acting.

He was also less prone to outbursts and it took him longer to get to the pitch where he would explode. His activity level, though still higher than the average eight year, was nevertheless lower. This meant that he could sit in one place longer, either to watch television, read or draw. In turn this gave him satisfaction when he had a piece of work to show at the end of it. His time in the past had been spent destroying things, not creating them. We didn't have to tell him off so much and this had a ripple effect. The medication took the edge off his difficult behaviour and the result of this change made him less restless, less aggressive and more reasonable. He achieved more, had more successes, and this in turn gave him more confidence and on it went.

We bought him his first bike. Mind you, we still had to keep a sharp eye on him because of his impulsiveness. On one occasion when we had allowed him out on his vehicle, I heard hysterical screaming outside. I found him staggering up the road toward the house wailing and with blood pouring from his head. I cleaned him up, went and got the bike, and took him off to Casualty again. He wasn't too badly hurt, but he said he had lost concentration, fallen off, and hit his head on the kerb. For a while after that he stayed at home.

The next time he rode it was when his grandparents were visiting. Simon was ready to run them home in the car when to Simon's horror, Joey hurtled out of an alley on his bike straight onto the road in front of the car. Aside from Mum's near heart failure, Joey was all right, but this type of thing had to be watched out for constantly.

Medication for an ADHD child cannot, of course, turn a monster into an angel overnight. The long years of negative behaviour patterns, the time lost through school expulsions and even doctor appointments add up to a child who may be desperately lonely and almost undoubtedly with low confidence levels. Joey could not be trusted yet, as he had not really learned how to be sensible. He remained immature emotionally and behaviourally despite being quite a bright little boy. Though we still had a long way to go, our home life was certainly calming down. Any improvement was an improvement to us, and though he continued to display temperamental extremes, these occurred at a lower level. So even though there were still chaotic days when nothing seemed to satisfy Joey, and we still could get frustrated with him and shout at him, perhaps even giving him the odd smack, the changes in Joey were mirrored in changes for me too.

I was now ready to move forward. The first thing I did was to obtain as much information about ADHD as I could. I read up on how the brain works, the causes of ADHD, and books on effective discipline and parenting techniques. I began to have more confidence in my decisions regarding Joey. I began to trust my own belief in how I might ideally expect my child to behave.

This was something I had been unable to do previously, because his own confidence had been so eroded over the years and I always felt so sorry for him that I tried to make things right for him all the time. This had not given Joey the consistent boundaries he needed, and in hindsight it did not help him.

I set out a framework for myself with certain desirable behaviours that I wanted to encourage Joey to attain, such as taking in an inside voice instead of shouting all the time. This I trained him to do by repetitiveness. For example, as soon as his volume level started to rise, instead of screaming at him to stop, I would calmly say "Joey, please talk in an inside voice" and this I would repeat over and over again until he got the message. This is far more effective than asking an ADHD child to stop doing something, because in the new framework you should supply the child with the actual thing you want him to do. Instead of saying "Joey, stop bouncing on those cushions" a better alternative would be "Can you sit on the couch quietly, please." It didn't always work because there is no absolute consistancy with these kids. Everything is hit and miss, therefore sometimes it had an effect and he would cooperate, other times he would not.

There are all sorts of techniques like this, and they did work to some extent. It was extremely useful to read about the disorder, the effects it had on the sufferer, and examples of the bizaare behaviour which could be expected from those with this neurological condition. I was determined to do the very best for Joey that I possibly could. Firstly, he was owed due to all the times I lost my temper with him and got frustrated and angry with his inabilities. Secondly, I still felt guilty at the way I had let teachers and other professionals fob us off and pass by without offering the help that was so obviously needed. This was the aspect of things which I have found hardest of all to let go. I cannot forgive easily, and I still had much pent up resentment and anger at all those wasted years and felt for the emptiness of Joey's lost childhood. If things had gone on as they seemed to be going, I would have been looking at a second broken marriage, maybe a breakdown. Joey might have carried out his threat to commit suicide, or he might even have carried out some impulsive and violent act which would have wreaked havoc and ended up with deep trouble for everyone.

11

The Support Group

Holding the piece of paper in my hands, finally, that confirms Joey's ADHD, is strange, strange, strange. There in black and white signed at the bottom by the specialist is the diagnosis which can also let my guilt recede. I have a child with a disability. I was not a bad parent. I now knew that I was no more to blame than any other parent of a child with a physical or mental problem. I was overcome with a mixture of relief and anger. The anger, as I have said so many times, was due to all those wasted years. I began to get my head and ideas together, though, as the days went by, and the medication was keeping Joey on a fairly even keel.

There are certain accommodations that can be made to help ADHD children. The first one is acceptance. You can then stop forever asking yourself why? the condition is there, your child has it, and there is little more to be said. It is incurable, although it is manageable to some extent. The next thing is to educate yourself and your child (if he/she is old enough) as to what the condition is, what causes it, and how you can alleviate the stress and knock on effects of it. I pored over every book I could find on ADHD and the more I learned about it, the more everything slipped into place.

I began to forgive Joey, even though he could still drive me up the wall sometimes. I accepted that he had a disability and should be looked on in no worse terms than anyone with a physical disability. It was a liberating feeling however to find good points in Joey and then to encourage him, for actually anything. If he put his shoes on the right feet I praised him. And I stopped dwelling on his mistakes so much. When we had an altercation, I would correct him, then forget about it. By doing this, Joey was not carrying round with him the burden of guilt for all the things he did, and I was not carrying around a festering and growing burden of hate for his behaviours. We took one incident at a time. Slowly he began to trust me and did not take his anger out on us so often.

Diary
Good grief, Joey has been delightful today. He got up all smiles and said good morning to Simon. How wonderful. I feel really close to him when he is like this, and I could just hug him to bits. Days like this are few and far between though. After school he told me that he had been mentioned in Praise Assembly so he was also in a good mood about that. He went up to bed in the evening very pleasantly and without any arguing for once, settling down in his bedroom without fuss. Oh, if only....

I rang the National Support Group again to thank them for all their help and the referral to the right consultant. I told the lady that thanks to the radio program, her advice on the telephone, and books that I was reading, we were at last getting Joey sorted out. We talked about how familiar our experiences were, that thousands of other parents were going through the same thing. She asked if I would consider setting up a Northern Support Group and encouraged me to go to the newspapers and tell my story, expose our struggle and give inspiration to other parents still battling with the powers that be, to get the help they need.

My mettle up, I called all the local newspapers not really thinking they would be interested in my story, but they jumped at the chance to interview me. I spoke to reporters from various local newspapers and then the Yorkshire Post saw one of the features and they range me for an interview. The articles came out well, and the response was incredible as soon as they came to print! Little did I expect the effect of these would have on local people. My telephone starting ringing, and ringing, and ringing...

The West Yorkshire ADHD Parent Support Group was born.

Calls came with regularity from other desperate parents wanting advice. In a few short weeks I had a long list of families who were struggling in the same kind of situation that we had. ADHD is not rare, and appears everywhere. I learned more and more about it in order to pass on information to other parents. The impact of my published articles surprised me mainly because I was not prepared for the deluge of horror stories that other parents had to tell. I had thought we were the only family to be let down so badly by medical and education professionals. Not so! Some mothers rang in tears to tell me that their children were suicidal. Some had children who had grown up without help and were now on the streets after falling into the downward spiral of school exclusion, anti-social behaviour and even criminal behaviours. Some had sons in prison, and daughters behaving promiscuously. Parents were absolutely desperate and looking for help and advice. It seemed like in a short space of time I became something of a guru. I did my best to help and passed on my experience, and the school doctor even christened me 'The Mother of ADHD'. It seemed as if all of a sudden the whole world and their dogs wanted to speak to me.

A researcher from the BBC show, Kilroy, who were then doing a discussion on ADHD, rang me offering a chauffeur driven car to take me to Teddington and back if I would appear. The filming was the next day, however, and it was impossible for me to go. But, when the program went on air the following week my phone went mad again, and the snowball of calls began to roll, not just in Yorkshire, but from all over the country. The BBC had such a huge response from the program that a second show was recorded, and my calls continued. The phone rang morning, noon and night and some times as soon as I replaced the receiver, another call would come through. I was exhausted and realised that it was having a detrimental effect on me personally. I wanted to help, but the weight and absorption of others emotional strain along with my own, was more than I could handle.

I often wonder, now, what would happen if parents of children with cerebral palsy, asthma or any other condition were pilloried in the way that parents of children with mental disabilities are. There would be an uproar. Yet it is still though perfectly acceptable and even the norm for more fortunate parents and many professionals in various sectors to parent-bash and look upon ADHD as something which results from bad parenting or dysfunction in a family. Psychiatrists say things like "We like to look at the whole family" but when a child presents with any other medical condition, doctors don't say they need to look at the whole family. This would be ludicrous.

In my researches into ADHD, since Joey's diagnosis, I find we are currently in an unfortunate situation in Britain. There is strong resistance by professionals to educating themselves about ADHD and much reluctance to admit their knowledge is sparse or non-existent. They still readily pin all behavioural problems on psychological circumstances and prefer for nurture to have much more to do with this condition than nature, perhaps because the context and environment of the sufferer gives them something to do. Admittedly, surroundings can affect and also can hinder the management of ADHD but the condition is considered to be hereditary, and definitively hereditary, something our British 'experts' disregard at present.

Diary
My head hurts. I must have taken a hundred calls this week. I want to help other parents — I really do, but sometimes I feel so helpless and I often feel that I want to talk to somebody about my own problems. I need to dump those too. Not only the problems with the support group, but with our general situation with Joey. I too have an ADHD child, and although I did set myself up in this position, I feel some days that I cannot give any more. I need someone to give to me. I need to offload too....

Some days I would just crash into bed exhausted after speaking to frantic mothers who were being made to feel bad about their parenting, or who had been informed that their children had probably been subjected to sexual abuse, to fathers who couldn't seem to instil any moral values into their children and who were fighting to keep them in school because they had been excluded. I advised them as best I could, sympathised and empathised. ADHD is believed to affect one in twenty children, so on average there is at least one sufferer in every classroom. In the States and Australia ADHD is accepted and has been treated

86

successfully with medications for years, however Ritalin is not the only effective medication for this disorder. Nevertheless, at present, it is largely the only one many practitioners are willing to prescribe.

There are children whose parents are told that they have learning difficulties, but the diagnosis go no further. Children are diagnosed as dyslexic, but many also have ADHD at the root of their problems. Others have anxiety disorders or depression, but the underlying reason is not investigated or understood.

After making myself aware of how dire the situation really was both for sufferers and parents I began linking up with other support groups around the country. I soon had the West Yorks Support Group inaugural meeting organised. A phenomenal eighty five people attended the first meeting! A great number of the children of these parents were having educational problems of various kinds. Some were under threat of expulsion, some were already excluded, temporarily or even permanently, with no educational provision being made at all! Others were misunderstood and not getting the special educational and/or medical provision needed and to which they are entitled. Following the first meeting we got a funding grant to set up a carer's group and since then we have become well known in the area. We provide information to callers over the telephone, write letters for parents and advocate on their behalf when specialists intimidate them.

During this period I went on local radio twice, and went with some of the other parents down to the filming of John Stapleton's "The Time, The Place." In that first year we sent an immense amount of information out to parents and we encouraged them to pass it on to others. I also organised a large mailing to over three hundred schools in the area outlining what ADHD is, what causes it, and how to recognise it. Many schools then contacted us or referred parents to us whose children were having behavioural and concentrational problems.

We then ran a survey to find out about the quality of care available to families and sufferers. The results showed abysmally poor provision. It was apparent that where ADHD was concerned, the amount of help that they should be getting medically, educationally or in any other respect, was pitiful. Getting effective help was a lottery and to some extent still is.

Diary
Although Joey has been reasonable this week, we have had one or two horrendous days with him. He has started using one or two colourful words, which we certainly do not use around this house. The school is concerned that he is being abusive to dinner ladies as well as to teachers, so we are going to have to come down quite hard on him for this. Get your crash helmets on.

Some days later.

Joey has been terrible for the last couple of days. Although his medication is helping, it is not consistent. Joey still changes like the British weather, and as Dr. Green puts it well in his book Understanding ADHD: "It is like juggling Gelignite." I couldn't have put it better myself.
Joey simply does not comprehend the impact he has on his surroundings. He cannot understand how everything is interlinked, how actions have consequences. It is as if part of his thinking process is missing. It is like he sees himself in a vacuum. It is so frustrating, as this is why he doesn't learn. The understanding is just not there.

12

The Statementing Procedure

Even with Joey's improvements, he still required much help at school, and especially of a social nature. He was still unpredictable, could blow up at the slightest triviality, and was difficult to manage in a main classroom, if left unsupervised. Some of the other children were afraid of him and therefore he was somewhat isolated.

After I wrote to the Education Authority, reports were collected from the psychologist and a psychiatrist, the latter one whom we had seen some years before. The educational psychologist came into the class at intervals to observe Joey's behaviour. 'Statementing' took time, of course, but as weeks ran into months, barring one or two upsets, Joey continued to improve. Not dramatically, but little by little. We would have periods when Joey went mad for a few weeks but on the whole the good days were gaining on the bad ones. He went into his ninth year much better than he went into his eighth one, he seemed to enjoy his birthday, and took pleasure from his gifts which was unusual for him.

Diary
What a horrid day! From the minute Joey got up today, he was on the warpath. He has been completely over the top and extremely hyperactive. He has not been able to stick at one thing for more than ten minutes. First he went out to play then after a few minutes he was back in asking to go on the computer. This lasted approximately seven and a half minutes. He was bored already. He then got his roller blades on and went back out to play but after three minutes he was tapping on the window wanting a drink. Shortly after he was knocking on the window

again for something else and by now we were getting slightly edgy.
He then took the blades off again and went to his bedroom to
watch a video, but after another 10 minutes he was back again
saying he is bored. This cycle was repeated throughout the day and
by about three in the afternoon Simon and I were ready to blow
our heads off. Each time he came through the door he slammed it
and by about the thirtieth slam you are ready to box his ears. He
is so noisy. He would not dream of talking when he can shout, so
consequently Simon and I both have bad headaches again. I ended
up taking Joey to his Dad's earlier than usual because we had just
had enough!

Every now and again Joey would have brief periods of what I considered to be normal behaviour. For example, he would decide to save his pocket money in order to buy something bigger and more worthwhile. This seemed a major success because his ordinary attitude was spend as soon as possible and purchase any old cheap rubbish just for the buzz of spending money. But these times never lasted long and he would soon return to his insatiable ways.

As things improved however, I started to relax a little. Unfortunately, Joey then had a bad period at school which led to one week's exclusion during lunch times, which was extremely unwieldy and inconvenient for me because Emily was usually asleep around midday. I would have to wake her up to go and pick Joey up at lunchtime. Joey had also been having a few problems with some of the dinner ladies, so a week off at lunchtime gave us all a bit of breathing space. To commend the school though, after Joey's exclusion, they did not dwell on it. Much to my relief, they went on taking each day as it came. The Headmistress filled out a report about all the behaviours Joey was displaying, to go towards his statement of special needs.

While Joey regressed, the school team did their best to diffuse situations, and get him through the bad patches with support and confidence-boosting. You can read the Headmistress's report however, and understand that is is not easy for a school to deal with a child like Joey. All credit goes to them, however, because without the expertise of the teachers, Joey would not have done half as well as he has done.

'He was supposed to be sitting on the floor cushion but he was lying on his back pushing his fingers through a hole in his trousers. The teacher removed him from class and he was given work to do in the corridor. He refused to sit down and was running up and down the corridor, shouting and disturbing others.

Very disruptive in Physical Education making rude noises. After ignoring several incidents the teacher asked him to leave the hall and go to SNA. He slammed the door and did not go to SNA.

Hitting and kicking other children often as they are passing him. Very suspicious of classmates, always accusing them of telling tales. Continuously trying to rile other children so that he can retaliate.

Thumping a girl at the swimming baths. Making sexual suggestions with PE rope when made to sit out of country dancing. Writing swear words in his spelling book.

Continuously running in and out of school without permission, swearing at supervisor and telling her to F... off, nipping older girls bottoms, hitting, kicking and punching other children, open defiance, throwing chairs around the dining room and frequently swearing at other children.

He has no true friends. Many children are afraid of his violent behaviour. He seems to have no perception of other children's feeling or wishes.

When he is calm he can have a rational conversation on a one to one basis, but he can should very loudly and is unable to listen to what anyone else is saying. He immediately accuses other people. He cannot bear anyone to touch him or brush against him accidentally without accusing them of aggravating him.' [extract from the report]

Even with medication, the process for re-educating Joey into a normal way of functioning if possible, was going to be long and slow. The Headmistress specified a number of targets to aim for regarding his development:

- to lengthen Joey's concentration span so that he can keep on task for lengths of time appropriate to his age and abilities
- to develop social skills so that he can make positive relationships with peers and adults
- to distinguish between acceptable and unacceptable behaviour.

A behaviour program was then set up, and this has continued up until the present day.

Diary
I have felt so disheartened this last few weeks. Joey has been impossible. After building myself up to see the specialist and getting Joey on medication, I had thought my troubles were over or drawing to an end. I am coming to the conclusion though that they will never be over. I am never going to be free until I die. I wanted a cure for Joey and I believed I had found it but it is true what it says in the books. There is really no cure at this time. I am just hoping and praying that Joey will be one of those who grows out of this terrible thing when puberty hits. Apparently there are some sufferers who settle down somewhat as they get older. He is so hyperactive though. It is really difficult to realistically see this happening. It does not stop me hoping though.

I have been trying to get Joey organised. All his drawers are now labelled with 'socks' or 'shirts', etc. His mind is still in a total muddle where his clothing is concerned and I am trying to instil in him where his clothes belong in the drawers, and where his dirty clothes belong. He still seems to have a mental block where this is concerned. The boy can read so hopefully the labels will help him to sort this out....I am not holding my breath.

Although the Headmistress's report made it appear that Joey was completely off the rails, this was not strictly true. Her report was to illustrate to the Education Authority that Joey did need extra assistance. Aside from that however, Joey was improving. No shadow of a doubt. The new school had a great deal to do with this improvement because they consciously glorified his skills and good points and played down his deficits. They have done their job at school and left me to do mine at home. I have not been called in each day to hear what Joey had done that was wrong. They have coped and I have every confidence in them.

The statement of special needs eventually came through, stating that Joey would get full time assistance both in the classroom and at lunch time. This was the best possible outcome and I am convinced the extra help has been a major factor in the successful management of Joey's ADHD. Whether or not a parent agrees to have medication for their child, there are still other accommodations necessary at home and at school, in conjunction with the medication, to achieve the greatest success. Ritalin was lengthening Joey's attention span, enabling him to stay focused long enough to finish work. The assistant was employed to ensure primarily that he did not get into circumstances where he could not cope, therefore diffusing awkward situations before they got to a pitch where he would lose his rag.

Joey was assigned a qualified special needs teacher, Mrs. W., and they have always got on really well. She has a positive outlook and genuinely seems to like Joey despite his difficulties. No doubt she has seen other children with severe difficulties during her career so she didn't seem astonished by Joey's idiosyncratic ways. At Christmas he was included in the school play, the first he has ever been selected for, and this boosted his confidence no end. The new found belief in himself that the school has instilled cannot be measured, but now he even has one or two friends.

Obviously Joey was now improving in all areas. His class work improved to such an extent that it was on a par with other children his own age, and he even forged ahead in some subjects, such as maths and technology.

Really it was blips in his behaviour and responses that we had to keep an eye on continuously.

At home we also made strides and Simon was equally pleased at Joey's progress. They could communicate in ways not possible before. A new tease came in to our jargon, whereby Simon would say things like "Stop fussing, we're doing some male bonding". Many a true word is said in jest, and Simon felt delighted that they began to talk about football, electronics or men things. Simon had always been disappointed that he could not take Joey to football matches or play with him in the garden, due to Joey's temperament which would cause him to stomp off or throw a tantrum. This typical behaviour has made Joey a very poor team player over the years, and although even now Simon doesn't play football with Joey, at least they talk about it and discuss players and teams. Simon also started to make jokes about me and Emily ganging up on him, so that he needed Joey to go on the man's side with him. While doing nothing for the larger 'gender war', this made Joey feel valued and that his views were wanted and needed. This kind of confidence-boosting has helped in Joey's rehabilitation.

ADHD children need to be made to feel they are an important part of the family, but unfortunately until medication kicks in, it is often the case that everyday is a mixture of confusion, argument and chaos. So much time is spent saying no, and trying to stop unacceptable behaviours that there is often little room left for positive family interaction. On top of this, parents frequently reach the point where they cannot find a single positive attribute in the child, a tragic but nevertheless true feature of their family relationship.

Fortunately, with Joey, we were now able to recognise the things at which Joey was good and competent, and to encourage him in those. He is very interested in computers and electronics. He owns a little electronic kit which he uses to set up flashing lights, buzzers and alarms. All of this fascinates him. And he has also turned out to be quite a little artist. His drawings are very detailed because his co-ordination has improved remarkably since the medication. As for school work, the last report from his present form teacher showed that he is joint first in maths. The other kids also have a nickname for him, 'The Technology Whiz'! As he is also good in the subject and this is the first nickname Joey has ever had, it has made him feel more accepted by the other children.

Diary
At present a lot of professionals who our children come into contact with are totally ignorant about ADHD. They also have a strong resistance to educating themselves about the condition via the ten thousand publications world-wide about the disorder. Because of this, there are children like Joey, in children's homes, foster care, in prison and on the street.

These agencies must be made aware of how to recognise the condition and treat it, and be made to learn about the knock-on effects such as ruined family relationships, educational underachievement, conduct disorder and criminality, alcohol and substance abuse, depression and suicide. The condition is absolutely not rare and the devastation, both in wasted lives and waste of resources for society is incalculable.

Now this is what constitutes my work with the support group. Unfortunately there is still the opinion amongst the many so-called specialists that these children's problems stem from a lack of moral guidance. They insist that it is parental techniques and family dynamics which are to blame for the problems. There is also opposition from these same people regarding the medications for ADHD because of scare stories in the press based on ignorance and untruth. Unfortunately mud sticks. It is the support group's mission to tell the truth about this disorder and the issues surrounding it, and this is what I and other parents of ADHD children are doing. It is a long up-hill struggle but we must carry on.

We carried on, going to Jimmy's every few months, and over a period we have been seen by a number of the specialist's colleagues. We were made to feel very much at home and it was refreshing not to have to justify ourselves repeatedly to the consultants. From the time Joey was first diagnosed we faced a graded schedule of hospital visits: first every two weeks, then every four weeks and then we took him every few months. We all tried to keep positive and to look to the future with hope.

As I continued my work with the support group, we believed we had rescued Joey from a living hell, giving him hope for the future, and a modicum of confidence in himself. We were regularly contacted by families from all over Yorkshire and country wide. I encouraged parents to contact their local support groups if they had concerns about their children and I stressed to them that they should not continue to suffer in silence. ADHD is real, as any parent of such a child will tell you. Things will never be perfect we know and accept, and there will always be problems. But at a minimum some of Joey's difficulties have been alleviated, even if the fight was the proverbial 'by tooth and nail'.

What began to happen was that the self-same teachers, educational psychologists, school nurses and so on through whose hands we had passed in our struggle, in fact workers from all professions were coming to me via the support group for advice on spotting and treating ADHD. Joey's previous school doctor went on a course with one of the leading ADHD specialists in the country and set up an ADHD clinic in Castleford....so he did read the literature I gave him! He has stayed in touch with me regarding developments in ADHD and he once informed me that Joey was the first child he had ever seen with ADHD, but I suspect if the truth be known, that isn't true. ADHD is common. I can hardly believe that in a whole career in children's health, that Joey was the first case he had encountered.

The phone never stopped ringing. I felt that at last I was being taken seriously. It was becoming accepted that I did in fact know what I was talking about.

Diary
I have had many calls recently from professionals wanting information on ADHD, and have even had a call from a mother who was given my phone number from the health visitor. Yes, the same one I had battled with all those years. That really made my day!

I am giving a talk on ADHD to a group of nursery school teachers at their study day this morning, and this is a similar request to a number of others I have had recently. Speaking in front of a group makes me nervous, but Nikki from the Hyperactive Society is speaking too, so it will be nice to see her again. We had eighty five people to the support group inaugural talk at the town hall, so if I can stand up in front of that many, the couple of dozen people who I will be speaking in front of this morning won't be too bad I guess.

Joey is in one of his terrible moods this morning. He winds Emily up to such a pitch that she is shrieking, he is shouting, and my head is about to explode. It is 7.45 am. I asked Joey to go and get something and I got the usual backchat. I just don't need this grief at this time of the morning.

Joey threw a biro pen at me in temper; the nib hit me right on the tender skin on the back of my hand and a big lump appeared. It is extremely sore. I know a biro is not a heavy object but when hurled across the room at you it stings. I chased him to try and put him out of the room and up the stairs, but he is so strong (and now almost 5 ft. tall). We struggled as I tried to force him through the door. Roll on, school time!

Everything is so up and down at the moment. Joey keeps lulling us into a false sense of security. He will have a good, pleasant day, and then act like a complete moron the next. We don't really know where we are.

Oh, please, please, don't let him be regressing. Not after all we have been through, and the improvements he has shown recently.

13

Ups and downs: 1997

At the tail end of 1996 over the Christmas season, Joey was doing reasonably well. With the help and positive encouragement he was getting at the school we thought we were out of the woods. He had been getting "good work" stamps in his work books. Whereas before he had seen himself as different, odd, impaired and worthless, he now seemed to view himself in a class with the other children, and only needing that little bit of extra help. We still had problems, but seeming less than before. We tried to instil in Joey the fact that he is clever and always has been. This seemed to give him a measure of comfort. He stopped losing his temper quite so much although we accept that this is part of his temperament and he will probably always be highly strung.

We tried to boost his self esteem on a daily basis. This was a must. Every day I would tell him how proud of him I was and how I loved him and how smart he was (and must be to catch up to the other children in the way he had done.) This was not simple for me to do, because it was not always the way I felt. I could never have brought myself to say such things to him in the past, so this was a breakthrough for me too. But it did seem logical that if the negative drip of responses he had endured for so many years could have destroyed his self esteem, that positive reinforcement given in the same way should have the opposite effect. We would have to wait and see.

We tried to train him not to take everything to extremes, and to give the appropriate weight to situations by not over-reacting. For example, whereas if he had a disagreement at school at one time, this would spoil the whole day for him, I tried to help him see that this was only one incident in an otherwise perfect day. We also reminded him that even the most perfectly behaved child gets on the wrong side of the teacher sometimes. We tried to help him not take things so personally.

At least the family viewed the future in a more positive way. If Joey continued to improve at the rate he was doing, perhaps there would come a day when we would see him sit exams, and even pass them. We remembered a past when it was inconceivable that he could be expected to sit for three minutes, never mind three hours which such exams might take.

The school had what is called a Praise Assembly each week, and Joey would often get mentioned for smiling, sitting still or for playing nicely. The school really did a great job in supporting the areas of activity and attitude that they could tackle. We also tried to change our routines to accommodate Joey's particular patterns of behaviour. An example of this was in bedtime and bedroom behaviours. He had never been one to settle well, causing havoc with his crashing, hectoring for drinks, coming in and out. On Ritalin he did not sleep any better though he was going to bed calmer and could read or listen to music until his usual sleeping hour of about 11pm. Now that Joey was older, we let him stay up later anyway but we also compromised in that if he would stay in bed and read or draw then he did not have to try to get to sleep until he was ready. This seemed to work smoothly at the time, and it meant that we could put Emily to bed knowing that Joey would probably not wake her up with his noise.

Joey loves Emily very much, and her birth was a contributing factor to his development. He feels more stable with a sister who he can look after, and I have always encouraged Joey to take a part in Emily's life, from nappy changing to playing with her. He was always delighted when we allowed him to hold the tiny baby in his arms, and he felt encouraged that we had the confidence to trust him with her. He took on the big brother role with gusto and was very protective to her. The advent of Emily also took the emphasis off him as well. We had another topic of conversation then, and Joey was therefore left more to his own devices, feeling less pressure to try and conform to our rules. Luckily for us, he was improving, or so we thought.

Joey remained poor at keeping track of his clothes and especially his socks. He often went to school in odd socks, because I was trying out the natural consequences with him. We tried to strike a balance between encouraging him to make progress by himself and keeping him on perhaps too tight a rein. Joey did occasionally take some responsibility for his own things, and though his bedroom was still untidy, it was not as catastrophic as it had been before. Although he was still very disorganised I did have a pleasant surprise now and then, when I found he had tried folding clothes up before putting them away. I saw this as progress and began to think he might even start putting dirty washing in the basket one day.

Don't get me wrong. There were still plenty of bad days. Joey would still be giddy at times, and especially if he found me in a situation, like on the phone or with company, where I was not in total control. He would take advantage of these situations and get high and uncontrollable. But Simon and I were now reasonably confident about taking him out in social situations, unlike before. Joey began having pub lunches with us, and when he was specially good, he might be rewarded with a trip to the burger bar. How we had envied families for whom these types of trips were normal family activities. I also could go to a shop with him, or visit friends, mainly because my friends were from the support group and had ADHD children of their own.

Diary
Thank goodness Emily is not affected by Joey's unpredictable behaviours. She is responsive to instructions and actually strives to do what might be expected and waits for the approval in our voices and our reactions. Ask her to close a door or get something for you and she willingly toddles off to do it. She interprets the tone of your voice when telling her something is hot or dangerous....something which Joey never could. She also has a different genetic make-up of course, which lends weight to the accepted theories about inherited disorder.

Also by Christmas, 1996, the support group had grown so popular that Simon and I decided that I would have to slow down in my commitment to it. Calls were coming at all hours. Often we would be lying in bed at night about to fall asleep, and the phone would ring. Listening to Simon hiss about "the bloody phone ringing again" did not of course help. We even had a few calls in the middle of the night, so we got to the point of pulling the phone out of its socket after about 8pm. But still the calls bombarded me all day, and this on top of all the other support group work was beginning to get on top of me.

I felt unwell a lot of the time and, of course, I still had Joey to look after. My friend, Belinda, who had been with me from the inauguration of the group agreed to take over the calls along with two or three other members. It was the most effective way to go forward, by sharing the load, but I had to change my telephone number to make it happen. I also decided not to be involved in the meetings anymore, but I continued and still do to campaign for the cause of treating ADHD. I write a bi-monthly newsletter and numerous letters to Social Services, MPs and the other professions regarding the issues surrounding the condition.

By February, 1997, Joey had been on medication for approximately sixteen months. He had been having what he called bad dreams and bad feelings more frequently. He had suffered these occasionally since his encephalitis, but now he was also having frequent head and stomach aches. One morning he wasn't feeling well, but I had sent him on to school anyway. At about 9.30am the telephone rang and the teacher told me that Joey was ill and asked for me to collect him. I brought him home and settled him on the couch, only to become increasingly worried as he began to go a funny gray colour. I could not be sure but he seemed to be drifting in and out of consciousness as he snoozed. Suddenly I heard a burbling noise and when I looked up, he had froth coming out of his mouth. I shook him but he was unconscious.

Immediately I called for an ambulance, and as Joey came round he vomited all over the floor. He was rushed into hospital where he had a major fit. I panicked and was so distressed at these developments. He came round, but as he was being admitted to the ward, he went into another fit. I couldn't believe it. What was happening?

Would he survive? Would he be the same when he got better, or would he be put back again? Questions, questions, and much confusion.

Unfortunately for us all, not only did the fits unsettle Joey emotionally but his temperament and moods seemed to be affected for the worse again. Though he recovered sufficiently to come out of hospital, the rest of 1997 was a nightmare. Joey became stroppy, argumentative and even destructive again. One day I went into his bedroom to find that his pine bed base was cracked completely through. He admitted that he had been bouncing on it repeatedly, but it never occurred to him to mention that it was cracked to us. Simon went mad, of course, because we could ill afford to replace the bed at the time, especially as lots of other things in the house were broken or in their final days. To try and make the point to Joey, we made him sleep on a blow up mattress for a while until we could get the money together to replace the bed.

Things were decidedly deteriorating, and in summer we asked the specialist to refer us to the psychologist at St. James' because we were frightened that Joey's temper and aggression were becoming uncontrollable. We attended for a number of sessions and at each one, Joey just swizzled round in the chair during the whole of the appointment, spitting out expletives and behaving in a totally anti-social way. One week when we knew we were going to see the psychologist we recorded Joey's tantrums and our family's interactions on a cassette tape and took it with us. When we played it to the doctor, I don't think he could actually believe it. There was nothing but swearing, snapping and arguing on it. The recording made us appear completely ineffective as parents because we simply could not contain Joey's offensiveness.

Diary
Simon, Joey and I have been having sessions with the psychologist lately, and discussing new strategies for dealing with Joey's aggression and the problems he has in getting along with other people in general. Using the program suggested to us, we are reacting differently to Joey's tantrums and this is alleviating the stress a little for us. The only trouble is that Joey's problems are not confined to our house. The school situation is up and down at present and with the best will in the world, changing our reactions to him won't change his attitude to the rest of the world in any way.

We are being really calm now whenever possible. This really phases Joey. Simon is managing the situation far better than me, but then he doesn't look after him for such long periods as I do. Simon is reasonably fresh when dealing with him, whereas I have usually been with him for hours and find myself irritable most of the time.

Joey has been having some fairly difficult periods still, like when he head-butted a wooden door about fifteen times. We just looked at him and let him get on with it. I wouldn't be surprised if he didn't have a stinker of a headache, and maybe that will make him think twice about doing it again. But maybe not?

The theory behind the method we are using currently, is not to give Joey any attention for negative or inappropriate behaviour. Hopefully he will get the message that he won't get a rise out of us for such actions. It remains to be seen whether or not this will have any effect in the long run, as, after all, we have tried this in the past to no effect....

The doctor advised not to argue with Joey or to get pulled into his hypothetical arguments. We tried to follow this advice to the letter, but things did not improve. We felt we were really wasting our time with the psychologist, because management strategies, though they can help the family get on together in the home, cannot affect what happens when the sufferer is out of it. At school, in the street, or in social interactions, we could change ourselves, but we just could not affect Joey's behaviour. Finally these appointments were abandoned. Another 'specialist' bit the dust.

I wrote a long and heartfelt letter to the clinical specialist who first put Joey on Ritalin, and pleaded with him to try Joey on another medication. I wanted to try something called Clonidine because I had heard that this might combat some of his symptoms, the aggression, his tics and the hyperactivity at night, all of which were increasing. Clonidine is a medication given to children with Tourette's Syndrome, but when our appointment came around he would not administer Joey with anything else but Ritalin. Due to the previous year of problems, however, we no longer had faith in any beneficial effects for Joey. After more pleading the specialist asked a psychiatrist colleague to see Joey as a favour, with the hope that he might be able to come up with something.

Diary
A call from the school today. Joey has kicked or thrown another child's shoe onto the school roof. The caretaker got up the ladder to try to retrieve it, but it was no good. It could not be reached. I went into school at 3.30 and the headmistress asked me if I could pay for a new pair of schoes for the other boy. No way!....Joey would pay. He did not think much of this plan, and threw an enormous tantrum. If we make him pay it out of his pocket money then maybe it will teach him? It is decided that he will pay £1 per week for eight weeks and the school will pay the remainder from funds. I agreed to that.
As soon as I got home, the phone rang. The boy's dad got up onto the roof himself and got the missing shoe. Joey is off the hook....jammy swine!

Meanwhile things were going from bad to worse at school. Joey was excluded for a couple of weeks over lunchtimes. What were we to do? It appeared that at 10½ years, Joey was back to where he had started when

I had first started searching for help. He was older yes, but he had not matured. If anything, because of his size in relation to his behaviour, things were worse than they had ever been.

One of my support group colleagues from another area informed us that we might be able to get financial help from a charity which aids families of children with severe physical and mental disabilities. An application was put in and one of their workers came out to visit us. We showed her the bed that Joey had destroyed, and the three piece suite which by now was almost completely ruined with Joey's constant bouncing on it. She told us that there were funds available for replacement furniture, recreational equipment, clothing allowances and travelling expenses. This was such welcome news, because frankly we were going broke with Joey's destruction, his loss of clothes and equipment, and all the going back and forth to Leeds for appointments. And because Joey could not travel on the school bus like other children, there was the normal day-to-day ferrying back and forth to school. As we live in a village, the school is two and a half miles away from our house, and so I was doing up to fifty miles travelling back and forth to school, and sometimes double in the weeks when he was excluded. We assured the charity worker that help with some of the petrol expenses would come in very welcome. Although it is humiliating to ask for charitable help, we felt at this particular time that we had no choice. Although Simon has always worked, having a child like Joey puts paid to any career plans I might have had. In any case, we were left with the impression that we would be receiving some assistance with our needs.

Unfortunately we were sadly disappointed in our expectations. A couple of months later we received a letter saying that in their opinion, Joey 'wasn't severe enough' to qualify for help. I really couldn't fathom it at all. Even after Joey's long and convoluted medical history, we were still be thwarted in our attempts to gain acceptance for the severity of our problems. It was unbelievable and felt like a completely unwarranted kick in the teeth. By this time however I had already taken on medical and psychological professions as well as educational authorities, so I was rather well versed in writing, well....stroppy letters.

Immediately I wrote to the person responsible for the decision and I wasn't very polite. I thought that if we were not going to receive any help, I might as well vent my anger, and let them know what I thought about this kind of 'long distance' vetting (despite the visitor!) Getting my feelings off my chest made me feel good even if some people will say I am a stroppy cow. Frankly, I was past caring, and decidedly desperate.

Surprisingly, a few weeks later I got a very polite letter back with an apology for adding to my obvious distress, and offering to review their decision. I was asked to supply them with the documentary evidence that I could about Joey's condition and the names of the consultants that he was under at the time. They would then look into the matter further. Though this was somewhat of a breakthrough, I still felt angry that once again I would have to prove to someone how much we had suffered. Their worker had seen our wrecked house, and had even gone to school with me to pick up Joey on a day when he had broken some school property, so there was really no doubt about his awkward behaviour. Also I had told her about Joey's encephalitis and the fits he had earlier that year. I wondered how serious was serious? Or did they think we were lying?

Anyway, at least they were going to take a second look. I honestly thought that they would not reverse their decision, though I wrote back accepting their suggestion of a review. I then forgot about it, as one more lost chance of help.

About six weeks later, I danced around the sitting room when I opened a letter containing a cheque for several hundred pounds. The jubilation was not just because of the money; as much as this, it was the principle that Joey's condition and our suffering had really been acknowledged. Although I would never wish the hell on earth we had gone through on anyone, the experiences have been character building for us. We have become bloody good fighters in any case.

We replaced the smashed bed, and spent some of the money on recreational equipment for Joey. We were also allowed some money toward travel expenses and outings. Meantime, though this was genuinely of support, I was going through a lot of trouble with some of our neighbours. The trouble was as much to do with my campaigning and publicity as it was to do with Joey himself.

Unfortunately I have found that by having my face occasionally appearing in the local newspapers, and by doing interviews from which quotes are taken, there are always a few people, who for one reason or another, want 'to take you on' and bait you on the issues. This happened to some extent on the estate where we lived.

One parent in particular decided that Joey was just a bad boy, and it appeared that she gathered quite a few other mothers on the estate as well. Over a period of weeks, there were altercations with her. My usual pattern in such situations is to explain what Joey has been through, and how we have sought help, then to offer our information sheets and humour the complainant for as long as I can. But when the person comes to our door too regularly, usually with very minor peccadillos that Joey is supposed to have perpetrated, I get angry. I had just got this particular woman off my back with this method, when another mother took up where the first one left off, but rather less intelligently so. Quite a few times she came to our door over a short period. I was nice to her at first, but it got to the point where she was knocking at the door so frequently that I refused to open door. "Joey had thrown a stone, Joey had told someone to sod off, Joey had kicked back when her son had done something..." It was just plain boring.

One morning she came round to the door during a very stressful week, and she was shouting. Her son had done something to Joey (again) and Joey had kicked the boy's bike over. I was so fed up by this time with her whinging and moaning at the most insignificant things, that we ended up in a slanging match in the street. All the neighbours came out for a look as I backed her down the street the way she came, pointing my finger half an inch from the end of her nose the whole time. I gave her a few 'home truths' because, believe me, her son was no angel either. I literally screamed out about how she did not know us, or anything about our family. When she stated that Joey "shouldn't be allowed out" or that "he was never punished", she was being ignorant and spiteful. How did she know what went on behind our doors and in our lives?

In the end a big crowd gathered, and I'm afraid I just flipped. Simon said afterwards that he thought I was going to hit the woman. To be honest, I thought I was too, but somehow I didn't. From that day to this she has never come to the door again, surprise, surprise, and neither have any other of the mothers. So, one way or another.......

14

The Present Day

Our appointments with the latest consultant had been a total waste of time. We consulted with him over a four month period. He cut Joey's Ritalin down to half the dose at the first appointment and then took it alway altogether at the second. When I mentioned Clonidine, he, like our original consultant, did not want to prescribe it. He offered to go through the Connors rating scale tick charts with me and with the school authorities as well, but I refused. Why should we have to cover old ground? It all seemed ridiculous to me. He offered to refer me back to Castleford, I accepted, and so by December 1997 Joey was back to square one AGAIN. Now without a consultant, without any medication and with a referral back to a doctor from whom we had been discharged two years earlier, I didn't really know how to go on with any hope for the future.

Diary, Christmas Eve
I went to get the nine hour candles that I have been saving for christmas and find out that whereas there were three, there is now only one. Joey stole the candles because he said he "wanted to have some fun." I explained to him that his fun has now spoiled our fun. He is remorseful, but realise that once again he cannot see how his actions have affected others.He told me he had been burning them outside, and when I went around to the side door I found a big burned patch were he had been burning papers and the candles, right beside the wooden door. The house could have gone up!
Christmas day. Mum and Dad came around for dinner. We showed them where Joey has burned up the wall and the step.

What does my mother say? "Well, he couldn't set fire to anything on the concrete step, could he?" I feel like blowing my brains out....

The new bed which the charity fund had paid for less than ten weeks previously was now also broken. Once again it was broken in a place where it was impossible to mend. Joey was therefore paying for a replacement himself. We decided to get him a fold up camp bed that time, because he was not fit to have another proper new one. It was just a vicious circle. He paid us fifteen pounds out of his Christmas money and the remainder would come out of his pocket money on a weekly basis. Will this help him sort out the value and the purposes of money? We'll see.

Joey has been excluded from school over dinner times till the end of term. We are always back to square one. When I finally found out about ADHD and received treatment for Joey, I thought our troubles were drawing to an end. Almost two years down the line I realise that my struggle will never be over.

Ritalin has helped Joey, no doubt about it, and the educational accommodations put in place by the school have made a big difference too, but the problems in Joey's head go deep, and I have no idea whether or not we will all come through this ordeal. What will become of Joey when he grows up? His personality makes it difficult for him to form friendships, and the aggression and impulsiveness which is so much a part of him can get him into so much trouble...

Joey is just as bad as he ever was, only much bigger and stronger. We worry how he will cope at High School this coming September. We have looked at some special schools which might consider accommodating him. Our worry on this score was that if he was with children with perhaps even greater problems, his could well be exacerbated rather than helped. Academically he

111

is very bright, but his behavioural and social difficulties hamper him to such an extent that we cannot see how he is going to manage in the world when we are not there to help any more. I am also frightened that as he grows older he will intimidate us, and sometimes now I fear for Emily. He has injured her occasionally through accidents and temper.

Diary
Some of the time he is quite lucid and very pleasant. These periods can last from a day to a few weeks. When he is like this we enjoy him and try to teach him as much as we can in that short space, but then he goes off the rails again and we just cannot get through to him. He cannot grasp that his actions are not acceptable, that his actions affect others, and how they endanger him too. His actions are perfectly logical to him therefore as far as he is concerned the world out there is mad, not him.

Joey's hyperactivity has subsided slightly however, and I am hoping against hope that when puberty starts some of this problem behaviour will start to diminish. I remember saying and hearing that about the 'terrible twos' as well.

When you have come this far though, it is impossible to stop fighting and hoping. The children are there and our responsibility. Personally, however, I have to warn any parent reading through this account, that when you set off on the roads that I have been down, you must steel yourself for a fight. You come up against a brick wall of ignorance, you will be looked upon as neurotic, and you will become experienced in the fobbing off technique. You will encounter so-called specialists who are nevertheless not in line with or knowledgeable about current medical findings. You will often be intimidated, belittled and made to feel a failure. Your endurance will be stretched to the limit and you will sometimes feel that it is you who are going mad, slowly and painfully. You will encounter very seductive 'enemies' within your own family group as well, in the form of a parent or relative who rather than face the facts, continues to make excuses for your child. This cannot do your child any favours: when later, should Joey in a temper knife someone, it doesn't really matter whether or not the victim provoked it. It will still be on Joey's head, and you will still feel the shame and guilt of an ineffective parent. It is the hardest job in the world bringing up a child with ADHD, and it is not helped by the lack of knowledge and understanding of others. Maybe in the future when more awareness is raised, our children will get more help from the professions devoted to alleviating suffering. Until then we parents and sufferers can only struggle on, taking each day as it comes and praying with all our hearts for some relief.

During my eleven year quest to find an answer for Joey's problems I have consulted one health visitor, several General Practitioners, two psychiatrists, two clinical psychologists, one school nurse, the school doctor plus another school doctor who now oversees Joey's statementing, an educational psychologist and three paediatricians altogether. I have also tried Joey on Evening Primrose Oil, Ritalin and at one point a homeopathic remedy. Periodically we have also tried Joey on various dietary reforms, excluding individual items one by one, but to no avail. Not one of these have been able to help in a substantial way in the long run. It really does make you despair, at the same time as you realise that medicine is not an exact nor a perfected science. This is not a let-out clause for the medical profession and the least it should be is an enquiring set of minds who together are debating and discussing avenues for treatment for conditions which appear to be ill-understood.

Just what can you do? It is bad enough having ADHD in the household without all the other knock on effects of it. I just hope that any other parent reading this account will gain a measure of comfort in the fact that they are not alone. Although I have tried to illustrate the devastating effects of this terrible thing, it is impossible to fully understand the impact of ADHD until you have lived with it and through it. I hope that by writing this book I will have done my bit in raising awareness of the condition for the next generation of sufferers, thereby encouraging more research and more support to be devoted to the eradication of it.

15

The future?

Summer, 1998

Joey is eleven and a half years old. Although things have improved in certain areas such as schoolwork, his social problems remain pressing and oppressive. At times he appears to be making friends and reacting in more appropriate ways towards other people. But, we also have periods when he seems to go completely out of control again. Recently he has picked up some strange new behaviours. His habit of taking everything literally also is increasing and he is tending to argue every point, every issue, at every minute of every day. It is simply exhausting having to go round and round conversationally in circles until he is given an answer which is precise enough for him. Joey is pedantic, fastidious and obsessional. If the answer he is given is one he does not like, he goes on and on and on and on .... until you pray that he would just GO AWAY.

He has also developed a strange fetish: washing his hands many times in a day, not touching or going near certain substances or things. He becomes seriously concerned if there is the smell of bleach in the room and he worries about lead poisoning and anything 'toxic' (his words). He makes a tremendous fuss if anything touches his spoon or goes near his dinner plate, if Emily spills anything near him or if she coughs or sneezes within a certain distance of him. He resists using towels to dry himself, preferring to get the hairdryer out to dry his body, or to stand in front of a heater. If we try to instruct him or reassure him about these things, he throws one of his famous paddies.

First and foremost, Joey is still totally unaware of the impact he has on his surroundings. He perceives things differently from the rest of us. It is as if there is one rule for society and one for Joey. He simply sees life from a different perspective, i.e. his own. Having said this, he took S.A.T.s (Statutory Assessment Tests) at school last term and did extremely well! The science and maths exams were apparently especially easy for him. Generally he also appears to be getting on better with other children .... and teachers. He has started to have good words to say about his teacher and has actually admitted that although she is firm, she is fair. What's this? Reasoning at last?

We have had a couple of sessions with a new psychological therapist who seems to understand children like Joey. He has a way of boosting Joey's self esteem and working through consequences with him. The therapist also did some tests with Joey on audio and visual memory, block tests, shapes etc. This was to determine Joey's intelligence and his recall skills. The tests were for age 13-17 years old, and it turns out that

Joey's score in relation to his age went off the scale! He is literally in the top 1% of ability, possibly MENSA material and verging on the gifted. It is extremely difficult for us to accept the fact that a child who has had such severe behavioural problems can be so clever. If only he could harness this intelligence and subdue his difficult side.

In September, Joey goes off to High School and I have already visited and explained the extent of Joey's problems to the Headmaster. He is not at all phased. Perhaps this school is also going to be as good as the Junior School? We wait with bated breath.

Joey finished at Junior school four weeks ago, having missed the final week at school because of pains in his leg. He ended up having to go into hospital to have pins put in and his femur had come out of his hip. Ouch! Unfortunately for us, this has meant that an activity holiday that the Social Services organised for him in the school holidays had to be cancelled. Oh, how we were looking forward to the break! Joey will be on crutches throughout the whole of the summer holidays. Naturally this is both frustrating for him and extra work for us.

Earlier in the year a friend sent me a book on Cranio-Sacral Therapy which I had not heard of before. The technique sounded fascinating and apparently some practitioners have been able to claim great success with hyperactive and autistic children. I found a local practitioner and took Joey along for some sessions. Although he enjoyed the experience it did not appear to make any difference to his actual behaviour.

During the final term at school I was not called in for anything and there were NO exclusion threats. Joey's handwriting and numbers have improved remarkably recently too. It is really incredible, how much the look of his hand writing has improved in such a short time.

Some days we are reasonably happy with things. On other days, we feel helpless and hopeless again.

We saw a new paediatrician with Joey last week. Apparently all this is 'something more than ADHD' (his words.) Joey could be suffering with a co-existing condition which many ADHD sufferers do. The doctor has mentioned Asperger's syndrome (AS) which comes under the description of autistic spectrum disorders. This would certainly account for some of Joey's weird rituals, the way he takes everything so literally, his inability to recognise facial expressions, tone of voice and figures of speech and his very graphic and detailed way of drawing.

Simon and I have therefore decided that we would like Joey formally assessing on this count. If Joey does come into the autistic bracket (a much more acceptable and recognised label to general society) the help he will obviously carry on needing as he grows up may be more forthcoming than it has been so far. People know about autism; about ADHD the large majority of the general public does not.

What the future holds for us we dread to think. Sometimes we hope and pray, when Joey is having a good period, that his problems are declining, but something happens and our hopes are dashed again.....

Diary, 6th August 1998
Can anyone who hasn't lived with an ADHD kid ever really perceive the amount of stress parents like us endure every minute of each of our waking hours when these kids are around? Does the parent of a normal child have any inkling of what it's like trying to instruct, or negotiate with, a child who constantly moves the goalposts? Will paediatricians, psychologists or psychiatrists ever really understand that the problems we encounter with these children occur on a minute by minute basis – they are NOT isolated incidents dotted throughout an otherwise normal or peaceful day?

It is extremely frustrating for parents to have to pick out incidents or altercations to be analysed by these specialists because they don't occur in isolation. They carry on throughout the day, each one flowing into the next and compounding the original problem. Add to this the impact these children have on other family members, how they affect the overall dynamics of family interaction, the frequent school problems, hospital appointments and the rest, and you have here the potential for a lethal brew!

Here's what happened this morning when Joey came down:

"Hello Sunshine"

"Hello Moonshine," he replied. Oh Joey, why do you take things so completely literally?

He gets under the duvet which is covering Emily. They start minor fisticuffs so I ask him to move. He point- blank refuses, so we get into an argument and he tells me to F*** off. CHARMING! I fine him 20p from his pocket money for swearing (he's now at about minus £1.20 for this week) and eventually he calms down. I pass him a magazine to look at to try to get him back on an even keel.

"Here, Joey." He ignores me, so I repeat "here Joey."

"Eye, Mum, eye," he replies.

Again, he has perceived "here" as "ear." It is so frustrating! I know Joey has a problem but this is not a now and again thing. It is constant and frankly it gets boring to have to explain words, expressions and meanings the whole time. This sounds very unkind, but my nerves are worn down completely and just the amount of talking one has to do in a day explaining things or arguing is exhausting.

We then have the usual breakfast argument. In a nutshell he doesn't want any of the options I offer him for breakfast so he ends the conversation with "I'll not have anything then. I'll just starve!" Starve, starve! I've just offered him a larger breakfast menu than he'd get at the Hilton!

By this time I am starting to lose my patience. He gets up and goes to the door.

"I'm going upstairs," he snaps.

"Go on then. See you later," I reply nonchalantly.

Two seconds later he is standing behind me again.

"I thought you were going upstairs?"

"Don't see why I have to!" he screams.

Joey returns to his chair and then starts ragging his sister again. So I warn him that if he doesn't stop it I am going to 'count' him. This is where you use the 1, 2, 3 – then time out method. He hates this and it usually sends him into fits of rage. But what the hell do you do? "When you do that with Emily," he shouts, "she gets 2 and three quarters and 2 and nine tenths!" Oh God, here we go again. He tries to goad me into another argument with this. He's always doing this by either mouthing off, or saying something extremely emotive or offensive to family members or even teachers. He certainly knows which of my buttons to press that's for sure.

The time is exactly 8.45 am, he has been out of bed approximately 20 minutes and I am ready to scream. What a life!

Within weeks we shall be trying to prepare Joey and now his little sister for school attendance. On top of the everyday breakfast aggro we have to somehow get him into uniform with his lack of motivation to get ready and often his inability to even dress, wash himself or brush his hair/teeth. The poor planning and memory of ADHD children means that often books and equipment which have to be in school on certain days get left at home. It's like planning a military operation!

So anyone out there tending to have a suspicion that our children's problems are of our own making or who feel that maybe, just maybe, our parenting skills are at fault, remember that ADHD knows no boundaries. I pray for the constructive and sensitive support of teachers, health professionals, and even the general public in helping us face each day with some optimism. I have tried to relate the depths to which a mother like myself — and there are many of us — can sink in the face of the impenetrable wall of the theoretical future. ANYONE can give birth to a child like this.

It is bad enough having ADHD in the household without all the other knock on effects of it. I just hope that any other parent reading this account will gain a measure of comfort in the fact that they are not alone. Although I have tried to illustrate the devastating effects of this terrible thing, it is impossible to fully understand the impact of ADHD until you have lived with it and through it. I hope that by writing this book I will have done my bit in raising awareness of the condition for the next generation of sufferers, thereby encouraging more research and more support to be devoted to the eradication of it.

I dedicate this book to any other parent who has travelled these same roads, and those who are about to embark.

Appendix

Therapies believed to be of help in alleviating symptoms of ADD/ADHD:

Homeopathy
Cranio Sacral therapy
Nutritional adjustments
Natural supplements
Medication
Special Needs assistance in school
Home management techniques

Resources & support groups

The ADD/ADHD Family Support Group UK
1a High Street
Dilton Marsh, Westbury, Wiltshire
BA13 4DL
Contact person: Gill Mead 01373 826045
The Support Group UK offers confidential and sympathetic advice over the telephone, and organises countrywide lectures and talks by professionals.

Local ADD/ADHD Support Groups

Berkshire ADHD helpline: Linzee Whitaker
01628 412555

Cambridge helpline: Trina Rogers
01223 3132287

Cornwall helpline: Julia Haywood
01726 816596

Dorset helpline: Sheelagh Hawkins
01305 778538

Northumberland helpline: Gill Priest
01670 789086

South London helpline: Sue Warren
0181 769 1667

Suffolk helpline: Lea Potter
01440 704151

West Yorkshire ADHD Support Group
Contact person & helpline: Brenda Maw
01924 863212

York helpline: Bob Breen
01904 782556

ADD Information Services (ADDISS)
P.O. Box 340
Edgware, Middlesex HA8 9HL
Contact person: Andrea Bilbow
Tel: 0180 905 2013
FAX: 0180 386 6466
e-mail: addiss@compuserve.com
ADD Information Services supply specialist books, audio and video tapes by mail order. A catalogue is available on request. They organise training for professionals and parents and offer free information to telephone callers including referral to local support groups.

International Psychology Services (IPS)
17 High Street
Hurstpierpoint, West Sussex, BN6 9TT
Training and conferences
Tel: 01273-832181
FAX: 01273-833250
e-mail: adholcourse@ips.prestel.co.uk

Societies & organisations

(National) Autistic Society
276 Willesden Lane
London NW2 5RB
Tel: 0181 451 1114
Family advice line: 0181 830 0999

Autistic Related Syndromes Support Group
15 Kingsdale Croft
Stretton, Burton on Trent DE13 0EG
Tel: 01283 530557

Contact a Family
170 Tottenham Court road
London W1P OHA
Tel: 0171 380 1261
FAX: 0171 383 0259
e-mail: carol@cafamily.org.uk

Dyslexia Institute
14 Haywra Street
Harrogate, North Yorkshire HG1 5BJ
Tel: 01423 522111
Website: www.dyslexia-inst.org.uk

Dyspraxia Foundation
8 West Alley
Hitchin, Herts SG5 1EG
Tel: 01462 454986
FAX: 01462 455052

Hyperactive Society
71 Whyke Lane
Chichester, West Sussex TO19 2LD (SAE with enquiry)
Offers holistic approaches to the management of ADHD.

Parents In Need of Support (PINS)
HVDA, Rockhaven, Victoria Road
Hartlepool
Tel: 01429 262641
A voluntary support group offering practical and emotional help to parents whose children are, or may be about to become involved in crime.

Sleep Scotland
8 Hope Park Square
Edinburgh EH8 9NW
Tel: 0131 6503078
e-mail: SleepScotland@ed.ac.uk
Charity aiming to give help and raise the profile of problems that devastate families with special needs children who have severe sleep difficulties.

Support in the North
Offering advice and help to other support groups.
40 Ravens Crescent
Dewsbury, West Yorkshire
Tel: 01924 469892

Syndromes Without A Name (SWAN)
16 Achilles Close
Wyrley, Walsall, West Midlands W56 6JW
Tel: 01922 701234
Support Group for families with children who have undiagnosed/unnamed conditions.

Information on the Internet

ADDnet UK
The premier British ADD web site. Information, useful links and listings of the regional support groups and specialists. Regularly updated.
http://www.web-tv.co.uk/addnet.html

ADD Update
My own web site about The ADD Update, a bi-monthly ADHD newsletter I edit with information for parents and teachers. Book reviews, links and other resources.
http://www.gailmiller.clara.net

Addvance
*Re*source site for girls and women with ADD
http://addvance.com

ADD Warehouse
If you need a book on any aspect of the condition, you will find it here. Also videos, audio cassettes, worksheets, assessment products, newsletters. Free catalogue available.
http:/www.addwarehouse.com

CHADD
Large American Support Group. Lots of information on all aspects of ADHD. Classroom management, adult ADD and much more.
http:/www.chadd.org

Education World
"Where educators go to learn" Site devoted to all sorts of information relevant to educators of all kinds.
http://education-world.com

Hyperactive Children's Support Group
Holistic approaches to management of ADD/ADHD
http://homepages.force9.net/hyperactive

Institute of Psychiatry
http://www.iop.bpmf.ac.uk

Mediconsult
Excellent site on all aspects of health. Material for anyone wanting further information on mental health. Lots about ADD.
http://mediconsult.com/frames/add

The Mining Company
Extensive web site including information on ADD, plus information for teachers about managing ADD children in the classroom.
http://add.miningco.com

Parent Pals
Web site devoted to the issues of special needs education
Http://www.parentpals.com/index2.html

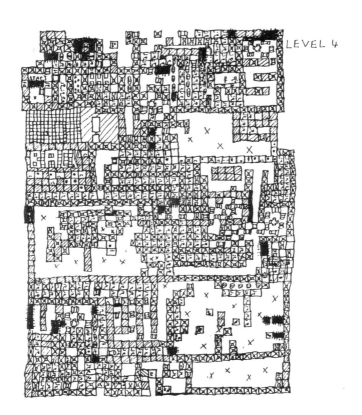

LEVEL 4